ENT AND HEAD AND NECK PROCEDURES
An operative guide

George Mochloulis, MD, CCST (ORL-HNS)
Consultant ENT and Head and Neck Surgeon
Lister Hospital, Stevenage, Hertfordshire, UK

F. Kay Seymour, MA (Cantab), FRCS (ORL-HNS)
Consultant ENT Surgeon
St Bartholomew's and the Royal London Hospitals, London, UK

Joanna Stephens, MBChB, FRCS (ORL-HNS)
ENT SpR
Royal National Throat Nose & Ear Hospital, London, UK

CRC Press
Taylor & Francis Group

CRC Press
Taylor & Francis Group
6000 Broken Sound Parkway NW, Suite 300
Boca Raton, FL 33487-2742

© 2014 by Taylor & Francis Group, LLC
CRC Press is an imprint of Taylor & Francis Group, an Informa business

No claim to original U.S. Government works

Printed on acid-free paper
Version Date: 20130801

International Standard Book Number-13: 978-1-84076-196-2 (Paperback)

Visit the Taylor & Francis Web site at
http://www.taylorandfrancis.com

and the CRC Press Web site at
http://www.crcpress.com

Contents

Contents

Preface

There are a number of excellent operative textbooks available, which provide detailed specialist and subspecialist knowledge. However, we feel there is a need for a clear, concise, step-by-step operative guide, to which the junior trainee can refer for an overview of core Otolaryngology, Head and Neck, and Facial Plastics procedures. This book hopes to provide comprehensive information to allow the trainees to perform the operations themselves under appropriate supervision, and is designed to be small enough to carry with you day to day.

As a team of authors, we have drawn on our experience, both at trainee and consultant level, and from colleagues within the specialty to put together a practical guide of how to make an operation succeed. Although different surgical approaches can provide equally good outcomes, this is beyond the scope of this textbook. We have simply described tried and tested techniques, which we find work.

Similarly, while we have included an easy reference table of complications that should be discussed with the patient when obtaining consent, we have not included a discussion on the surgical anatomy, indications, or benefits.

We are extremely grateful to our coauthors, and would like to thank them for their help and contributions, as outlined below. In addition, special thanks go to Nikos Papadimitriou for his help in the early stages of writing, and to Alasdair Mace for his invaluable help with reviewing this book.

Contributors

5 – Mr. S. Ahluwalia
5 – Prof. A. Narula
6 – Mr. C. Giddings
14 – Mr. A. Frosh
15, 16 – Mr. C. Georgalas
23, 24 – Mr. K. Ghufoor
34 – Mr. N. Tolley

Consent Table

Otology	Bleeding	Infection	Chronic otorrhoea	Residual perforation	Scar	
Chapter						
1 Grommet insertion	√	√	√	√		
2 Excision lesion pinna	√	√			√	
3 Excision preauricular sinus	√	√			√	
4 Myringoplasty	√	√		√	√	
5 Ossiculoplasty	√	√			√	
6 Stapedotomy	√	√			√	
7 Mastoidectomy	√	√		√	√	

Rhinology	Bleeding	Infection	Septal perforation	Scar	Nasal obstruction	
9 MUA of fractured nose	√				√	
10 Septoplasty	√	√	√		√	
11 Surgery to inferior turbinates	√	√				
Surgical management of epistaxis:						
12 SPA ligation +/- septoplasty	√	√	√			
13 Anterior ethmoid artery ligation	√	√		√		
14 Endoscopic sinus surgery +/- septoplasty	√	√	√			
15 Septorhinoplasty	√	√	√	√	√	
16 Lateral rhinotomy and medial maxillectomy	√	√	√	√		
17 Maxillectomy	√	√		√		
18 DCR +/- septoplasty	√	√	√			

Head and Neck	Bleeding	Infection	Scar	Tracheostomy	Nerve injury	
21 FNAC	√	√				
22 Lymph node biopsy	√	√	√		XI; marginal mandibular	
23 Tonsillectomy and adenoidectomy	√	√				
24 Uvulopalatoplasty	√	√				
25 Tracheostomy	√	√	√			

Alteration in taste	Dizziness	Reduced hearing	Tinnitus	Dead ear	Facial nerve injury	Further surgery
						√
						√
√	√	√	√			√
√	√	√	√	√		√
√	√	√	√	√	√	√
√	√	√	√	√	√	√

CSF leak	Visual disturbance	Further surgery	Nasal packs	POP		
		√	√	√		
			√			
			√			
√		√	√		√	
		√	√			
√	√	√	√			
		√	√	√		
√	√	√	√	√		
	√	√				√
√	√	√				

Dental trauma	Nasal regurgitation	Pain	Perforation	Recurrence	Further surgery	Drain
		√				
√	√	√				
√	√	√		√		
		√				

(Continued)

Head and Neck	Bleeding	Infection	Scar	Tracheostomy	Nerve injury	
Chapter						
26 Endoscopy – diagnostic procedures of upper aerodigestive tract	√	√				
27 Paediatric MLB and bronchoscopy	√	√		√		
28 Phonosurgery	√	√		√		
29 Microlaryngoscopy	√	√		√		
30 Pharyngeal pouch repair – endoscopic and open approach	√	√	√		recurrent laryngeal	
31 Submandibular gland excision	√	√	√		marginal mandibular, XII	
32 Parotidectomy	√	√	√		VII + sensory of great auricuar nerve	
33 Thyroglossal cyst excision	√	√	√			
34 Thyroidectomy	√	√	√		recurrent laryngeal & EBSLN	
35 Neck dissection	√	√	√		XI, XII, marginal mandibular	
36 Total laryngectomy + TEP	√	√	√	√	XI, XII, marginal mandibular	

Facial Plastics	Bleeding	Infection	Scar	Necrosis of skin/flap	Unsatisfactory cosmetic result	
38 Local flaps	√	√	√	√	√	
39 Pinnaplasty	√	√	√	√	√	
40 Blepharoplasty	√	√	√		√	
41 Face lift	√	√	√		√	

Note

Scar - may be normal/hypertrophic/keloid
CSF: cerebrospinal fluid
DCR: dacryocystorhinostomy
EBSLN: external branch of superior laryngeal nerve
FNAC: fine needle aspiration cytology
MLB: microlaryngoscopy and bronchoscopy

MUA: manipulation under anaesthesia
SPA: sphenopalatine artery
POP: plaster-of-Paris
TEP: tracheoesophageal puncture

Dental trauma	Nasal regurgitation	Pain	Perforation	Recurrence	Further surgery	Drain
√		√	√		√	
√					√	
√					√	
√					√	
√		√	√	√	√	√
		√				√
		√				√
		√		√		√
		√				√
		√				√
		√	leak			√

Incomplete excision	Nerve injury	Dry eyes	Ectropion/ entropion	Visual disturbance	Alopecia	
√	temporal, marginal mandibular					
		√	√	√		
	motor branches of facial, sensory				√	

1 Grommet insertion

SURGICAL STEPS

1 **Positioning the patient**
2 **Examination under the microscope**
3 **Myringotomy**
4 **Grommet insertion**

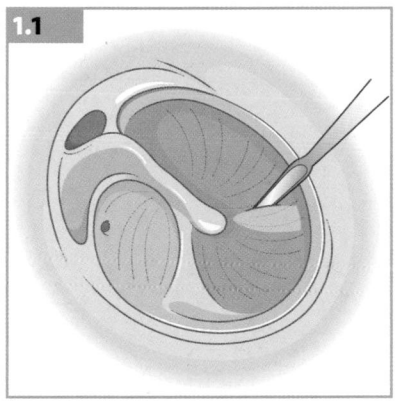

1.1 *The tympanic membrane.*

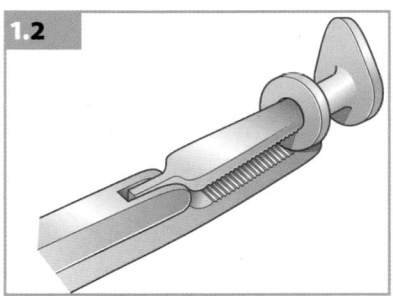

1.2 *Inserting the grommet.*

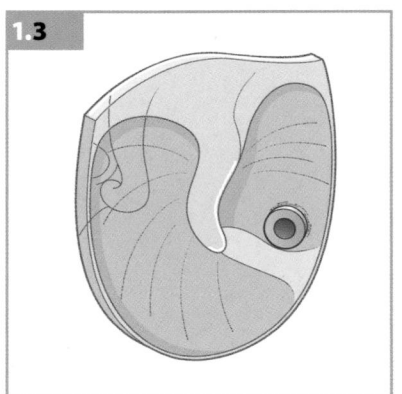

1.3 *Completion of grommet insertion.*

PROCEDURE

1 Positioning the patient
Position the operating table head-up. Turn the patient's head away from the operative side and position the aperture drape. ✪

2 Examination under the microscope
Clean the external auditory canal and inspect the tympanic membrane. Take care to avoid injury to the external auditory canal skin.

3 Myringotomy
Use a myringotomy knife to make a radial incision in the antero-inferior quadrant of the tympanic membrane (**1.1**). The length of the incision should match the diameter of the inner flange of the grommet. Any middle ear effusion should be removed using 22 gauge suction. ✪✪

4 Grommet insertion
Insert the grommet through the myringotomy incision using crocodile forceps (**1.2**). Complete insertion of the grommet using a slightly curved needle (**1.3**). Suction any blood or fluid from the grommet lumen. Instill drops to prevent blockage of the grommet lumen.

✪ ***Surgeon's tip***
If operating on a patient with Down's syndrome, take care with neck positioning as there is a higher incidence of atlanto–axial instability.

✪✪ ***Surgeon's tip***
Avoid touching the edges of the myringotomy with the suction tip as this may cause peri-operative bleeding and tympanosclerosis.

2 Removal of lesion from pinna – wedge excision

SURGICAL STEPS

1 **Positioning the patient**
2 **Draping and local anaesthetic**
3 **Excision of the lesion**
4 **Closure and dressing**

PROCEDURE

1 Positioning the patient

The patient is placed supine on the operating table, on a head ring. Turn the patient's head away from the operative side. Use a sterile marker pen to mark the resection margins (**2.1**). Commonly, lesions occur on the edge of the pinna, and a wedge excision gives adequate clearance and a reasonable cosmetic result. See *Table 2.1* for excision margins required for different lesions.

2 Draping and local anaesthetic

Prepare the skin with betadine, and use a small piece of cotton wool to prevent it entering the external auditory canal. If the procedure is being done under general anaesthesia, use a head drape; leave the face exposed if the procedure is being done under local anaesthetic. Inject 2–4 ml of local anaesthetic and adrenaline in the form of 2% lignocaine and 1/80,000 adrenaline using a dental syringe.

3 Excision of the lesion

Use a 15 blade to excise the lesion as marked, using a full thickness incision (**2.2**). Use a marking stitch (2/0 silk) to orientate the specimen for histology. ✪

4 Closure and dressing

Use 5/0 prolene to suture the skin edges anteriorly and posteriorly, making sure that the cartilage edges are completely covered. Use a paraffin impregnated gauze such as Jelonet® to fill the contours of the external ear and cover the postauricular aspect of the incision. Apply a head bandage.

Table 2.1: EXCISION MARGINS FOR LESIONS

Lesion	Excision margin
Simple BCC	2–3 mm
Morpheaform BCC	5 mm
Low risk SCC	4 mm
High risk SCC (i.e. diameter >2 cm or depth >6 mm)	6 mm
Malignant melanoma	Dependent on staging

BCC: basal cell carcinoma; SCC: squamous cell carcinoma

✪ Surgeon's tip

Once you have excised the lesion, excise a small ellipse of cartilage on either side of the wedge so that you may achieve an adequate approximation of the skin both on the anterior and posterior aspect of the pinna.

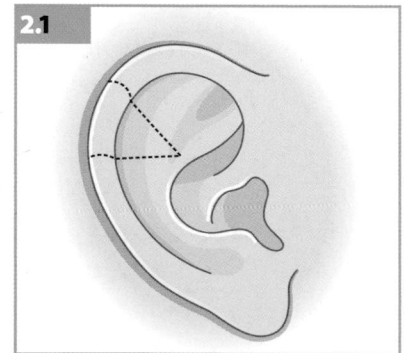

2.1 *Marking of pinna wedge.*

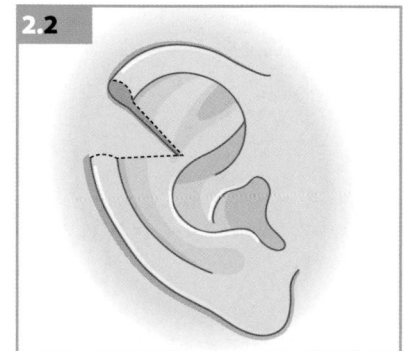

2.2 *Wedge excision.*

3 Excision of preauricular sinus

SURGICAL STEPS

1 **Positioning the patient**
2 **Examination under the microscope**
3 **Injection of methylene blue to define the sinus tract**
4 **Skin incision**
5 **Excision of the sinus tract**
6 **Closure**

PROCEDURE

1 Positioning the patient
Position the operating table head-up. Turn the patient's head away from the operative side. Mark an elliptical incision around the opening of the sinus. Prepare the skin with betadine, and drape the patient tightly with a head drape to hold hair out of the operative field.

2 Examination under the microscope
Examine the external auditory meatus under the microscope to exclude the pit of a preauricular fistula opening into the ear canal.

3 Injection of methylene blue to define the sinus tract
Using a blunt needle, gently inject methylene blue into the sinus. Probe the sinus with a lacrimal probe to determine direction and length of the sinus tract. Alternatively, a thick prolene suture can be used. Inject skin with approximately 1–2 ml of 2% lignocaine with 1/80,000 adrenaline. ✪

4 Skin incision
Using a 15 blade, make the skin incision following relaxed skin tension lines. Raise skin flaps anteriorly for approximately 2 cm, and as far as the perichondrium of helical cartilage posteriorly. Use an assistant to retract skin flaps with skin hooks (**3.1**).

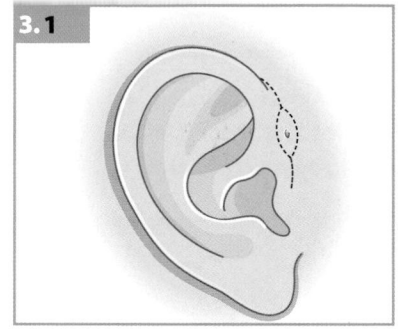

3.1 *Excision of preauricular sinus – marking the incision.*

5 Excision of the sinus tract
Retract an island of tissue around the sinus opening with Allis forceps. Using iris scissors, carefully dissect the sinus tract through subcutaneous tissues. Take care not to breach the walls of the sinus. If the fundus of the sinus is adherent to the helical perichondrium, excise a segment of cartilage with the specimen. ✪✪

6 Closure
Ensure haemostasis. Skin incisions are closed with 3/0 vicryl and 4/0 prolene and sprayed with a transparent dressing such as Opsite spray. No other dressing is required.

✪ *Surgeon's tip* _____
Take care not to damage the walls of the sinus with the probe or needle.

_____

✪✪ *Surgeon's tip* _____
A lacrimal probe can be placed in the sinus tract to help identify it when you are dissecting through subcutaneous tissues.

_____

✪✪ *Surgeon's tip* _____
Look for bluish colouration of methylene blue to highlight the sinus tract.

4 Myringoplasty

SURGICAL STEPS

1 **Positioning the patient**
2 **Examination under the microscope; freshen the edges of perforation**
3 **Surgical approaches:**
   - Postauricular
   - Endaural
   - Permeatal
4 **Harvesting the temporalis fascia graft**
5 **Elevating the tympanomeatal flap**
6 **Positioning the graft**
7 **Packing and closure**

PROCEDURE

1 Positioning the patient

Position the patient on a head ring with operating table head-up. Turn the patient's head away from the operative side. Shave the hair over the incision site. Inject approximately 10 ml of local anaesthetic and adrenaline in the form of 1% lignocaine and 1/200,000 adrenaline. Prepare the skin with betadine, and drape the patient tightly with a head drape to hold hair out of the operative field.

2 Examination under the microscope; freshen the edges of perforation

Using a microscope, clean the ear canal and assess perforation site and size. Inject 1–2 ml of 2% lignocaine and 1/80,000 adrenaline using a dental syringe. Inject slowly at the edge of hair-bearing skin, from 12 o'clock to 6 o'clock (**4.1**). Freshen the edges of perforation using a slightly curved needle to remove the thin rim of squamous epithelium from the perforation edge.

3 Surgical approaches
Postauricular

Using a 10 blade, make a skin incision 0.5–1 cm behind the postauricular sulcus, from the inferior margin of the external auditory meatus inferiorly to the level of the zygomatic arch superiorly (**4.2**). Continue the incision through the postauricular muscles to the level of the temporalis fascia superiorly. Dissect as far as the posterior edge of bony external auditory canal. ✪

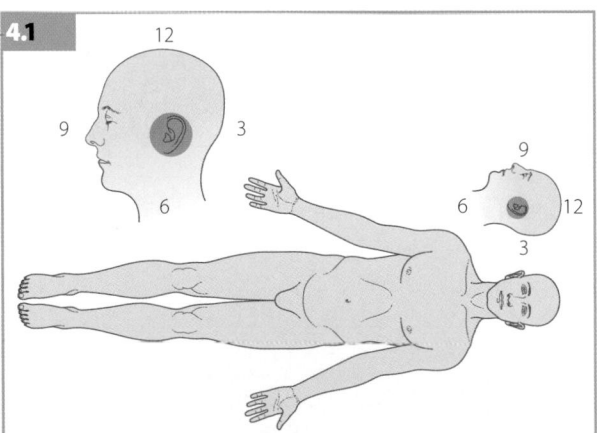

***4.1** Clockface used to describe positions on the tympanic membrane or ear canal.*

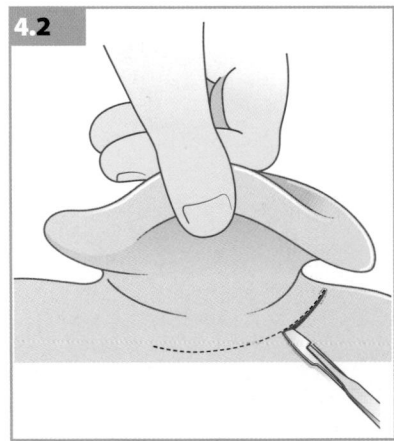

***4.2** Postauricular skin incision.*

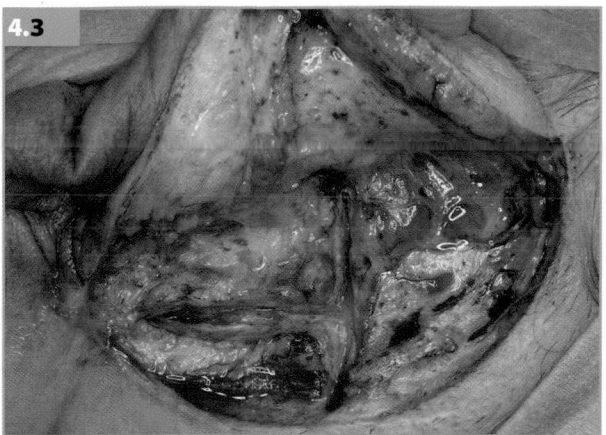

4.3–4.5 Postauricular approach to myringoplasty.

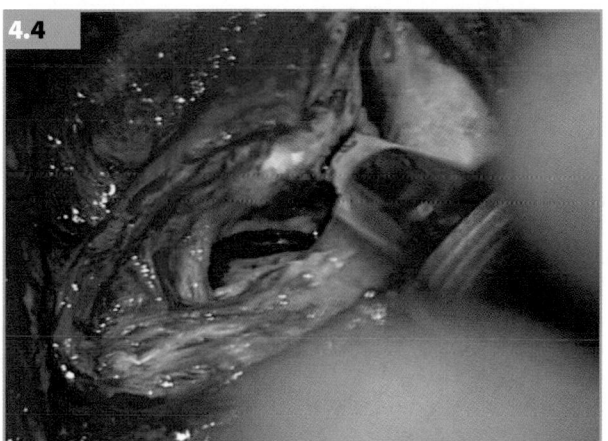

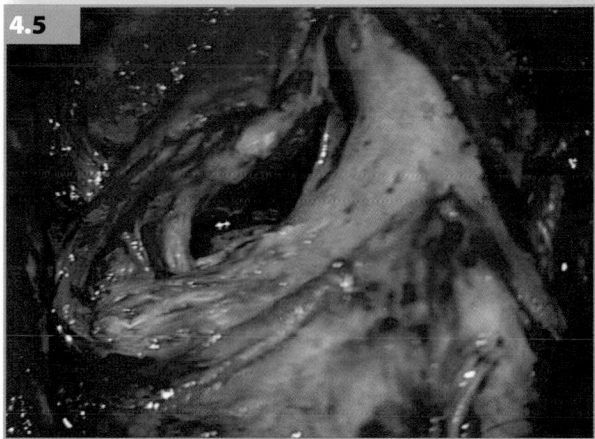

Using a 15 blade, make a T-shaped incision (**4.3**). Elevate periosteum with a Freer elevator, taking care not to tear periosteum or external auditory canal skin, especially at the spine of Henle. Enter the ear canal lumen using an incision through external auditory canal skin (**4.4**, **4.5**). Quarter-inch ribbon gauze is passed through the incision and the two ends held in a clip, retracting skin and pinna anteriorly. Insert two self-retaining retractors. ✪✪

✪ **Surgeon's tip**

Holding the pinna between thumb and index finger, with the index finger in the external auditory meatus, retract the pinna anteriorly. Using a knife at 45° to the skull, dissect anteriorly in this plane, as far as the posterior edge of bony external auditory canal. This avoids damaging the temporalis fascia or perforating the posterior external auditory canal skin.

✪✪ **Surgeon's tip**

If the full extent of the perforation cannot be visualised because of a narrow or tortuous external auditory canal, a canalplasty may be required. See 7 – Mastoidectomy and canalplasty.

✪ Surgeon's tip _____

To avoid damage, do not allow the suction tip to touch the tympanomeatal flap. Always suck behind the round canal knife, or through cotton wool.

✪✪ Surgeon's tip _____

To avoid damage to the ossicular chain and chorda tympani, start the elevation of the annulus in the postero-inferior quadrant.

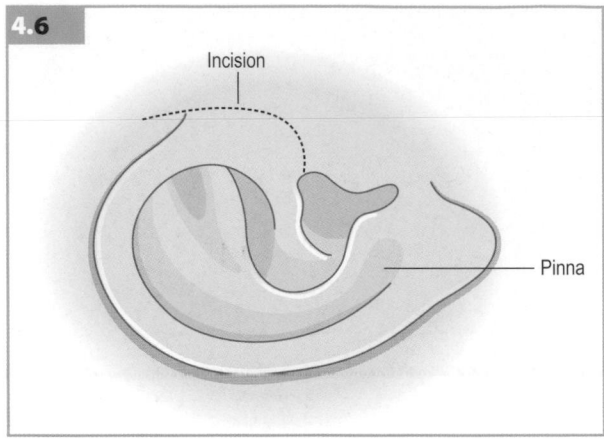

4.6 *Endaural approach to myringoplasty.*

Endaural

Using a 15 blade, make a skin incision between the tragus and root of helix, and extend superiorly over the zygomatic arch as far as the temporalis fascia (**4.6**). Take care to avoid damaging cartilage. Using a Lempert speculum, extend the incision deep through the periosteum from the level of the zygomatic arch superiorly into the roof of the ear canal for 5 mm. Insert two self-retaining retractors.

Permeatal

Make a single hairline incision to access the temporalis fascia and a tympanomeatal flap incision in external auditory canal skin.

4 Harvesting the temporalis fascia graft

Lift the scalp with a Langenbeck retractor. Dissect the plane above the temporalis fascia using scissors. Incise the temporalis fascia, and separate fascia off muscle with a Freer elevator. Using nontoothed forceps and curved iris scissors, harvest the graft (size appropriate to the tympanic defect). Spread the graft out on a glass slide to dry.

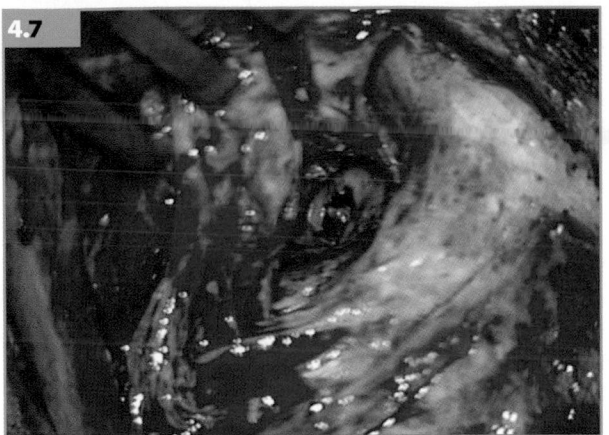

4.7 *Elevating the tympanomeatal flap.*

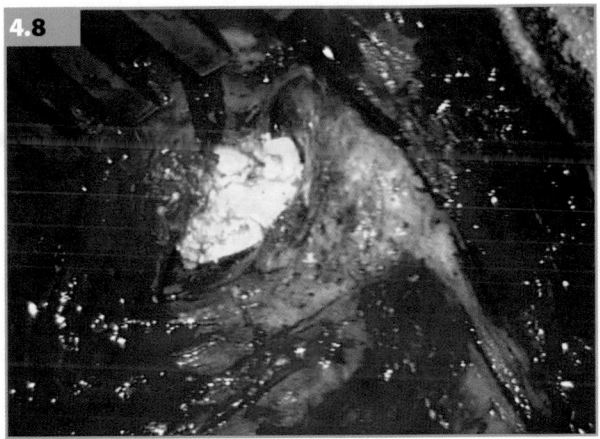

4.8 *Closure and packing.*

5 Elevating the tympanomeatal flap

Using a 45° round canal knife, make an incision 10 mm lateral to the annulus, extending from 12 to 6 o'clock. Use a Plester D-knife to make two longitudinal incisions as shown in Figure **4.7**. Use the round canal knife to elevate the tympanomeatal flap until you reach the annulus. ✪

Lift the annulus out of the annular rim using a flat canal elevator and use a slightly curved needle to enter the middle ear space. Elevate the annulus from 12 to 6 o'clock. ✪✪

6 Positioning the graft

Cut the graft to size. Holding the front edge of the graft in a pair of crocodile forceps, place underneath the tympanic membrane, ensuring that the graft covers the defect. Place some pieces of sofradex-soaked absorbable gelatin sponge in the middle ear to support the graft. ✪✪✪

7 Packing and closure

Pack the deep ear canal with pieces of absorbable gelatin sponge and bismuth iodoform paraffin paste (BIPP) (**4.8**). Skin incisions are closed with 3/0 vicryl and 4/0 prolene. A pressure bandage of paraffin impregnated dressing such as Jelonet®, gauze, cotton wool, and crepe bandage may be applied overnight.

✪✪✪ Surgeon's tip

Tragal and conchal cartilage are frequently used as alternative graft materials, especially when a stronger reinforcement of the tympanic membrane is required. If a postaural approach has been used, conchal cartilage is readily accessible. It should be thinned to a diameter of 2–3 mm using either a scalpel or cartilage cutter. Tragal cartilage is thinner and can be harvested via a separate tragal incision.

---

5 Ossiculoplasty

SURGICAL STEPS

1 **Positioning the patient**
2 **Examination under the microscope, tympanomeatal flap elevation**
3 **Ossicular assessment**
4 **Choice of prosthesis**
5 **Positioning the prosthesis**
6 **Packing and closure**

PROCEDURE

1 Positioning the patient

Position the operating table head-up. Turn the patient's head away from the operative side. Attach a facial nerve monitor and ensure it is working. Prepare the skin with betadine, and drape the patient tightly with a head drape to hold the hair out of the operative field.

2 Examination under the microscope, tympanomeatal flap elevation

Inject 1–2 ml of local anaesthetic and adrenaline in the form of 2% lignocaine and 1/80,000 adrenaline using a dental syringe. Inject slowly at the edge of hair-bearing skin from 12 o'clock to 6 o'clock. Using a disposable tympanoplasty blade, make an incision into the external auditory canal skin 10 mm lateral to the annulus, extending from 12 to 6 o'clock. Use a Plester D-knife to make two longitudinal incisions. Use a round canal knife to elevate the tympano-meatal flap until the annulus is reached. ✪

Lift the annulus out of the annular rim using a flat canal elevator and use a slightly curved needle to enter the middle ear space. Elevate the annulus from 12 to 6 o'clock. ✪✪

Fold the tympanomeatal flap anteriorly, identify and preserve the chorda tympani. Use the House curette or a 1 mm diamond burr to remove bone of the scutum if necessary to expose the incudostapedial joint (ISJ) and stapes footplate.

3 Ossicular assessment

Exclude any middle ear pathology. Use a slightly curved needle to gently assess ossicular mobility and continuity (*Table 5.1*). First probe the malleus and check ISJ mobility. Do not touch the stapes itself until this has been done. Secondly, assess the stapes footplate. Using gentle pressure on the ISJ, assess the mobility of the stapes. Is it fixed or mobile? Ensure at least 5 mm of middle ear space for reconstruction, particularly in post chronic suppurative otitis media cases. ✪✪✪

4 Choice of prosthesis

See *Table 5.2*, Figures **5.1** and **5.2**.

5 Positioning the prosthesis, e.g. PORP

Use a measuring rod to determine the distance that needs to be bridged and trim the prosthesis to size with a scalpel. Use fine crocodile forceps and the slightly curved needle to manipulate the prosthesis gently into place and achieve a snug fit. The prosthesis should sit comfortably on the head of the stapes. Malleus or incus should be placed onto the prosthesis making sure there is no deviation from the anatomical position. Assess continuity of movement.

6 Packing and closure

Check that the prosthesis is not resting on the tympanic membrane, to avoid extrusion of the prosthesis. If the malleus is absent, insert a small piece of tragal cartilage between the tympanic membrane and the prosthesis. Replace the tympanomeatal flap and pack with pieces of absorbable gelatin sponge and BIPP (*see 4 – Myringoplasty*).

Table 5.1: MIDDLE EAR FINDINGS AND TREATMENT OPTIONS

Likely findings	Treatment options
Fixation of incudomalleolar joint	Remove incus
Fixation of head of malleus	Remove malleus head with malleus head nippers
Erosion of LPI	Remove incus
ISJ discontinuity – post-traumatic	Re-establish continuity
Stapes footplate fixation	Stapedotomy

ISJ: incudostapedial joint ; LPI: long process of the incus

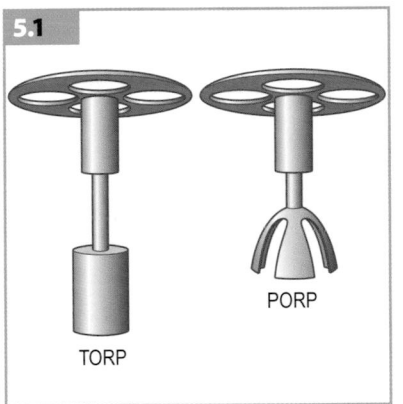

5.1 *Ossicular prostheses TORP: total ossicular reconstruction prosthesis; PORP: partial ossicular reconstruction prosthesis;*

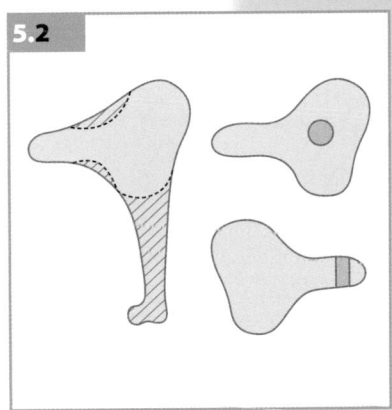

5.2 *Incus transposition*

✪ Surgeon's tip

No direct suction is used for fear of tearing the flap.

✪✪ Surgeon's tip

To avoid damage to the ossicular chain and chorda tympani, start the elevation of the annulus in the postero-inferior quadrant.

✪✪✪ Surgeon's tip

Beware a very narrow long process of incus, as this is probably a fibrous pseudojoint and will be compromised. If there is no ISJ, the stapes head may be fragile even if it looks normal at first inspection.

Table 5.2: CHOICE OF PROSTHESIS

State of ossicles			Prosthesis
Malleus	*Incus*	*Stapes*	
Present	Absent or eroded	Intact	Incus transposition *Or* Incus prosthesis *Or* PORP, bypassing malleus
Present	Absent	Only footplate present	Incudostapedial prosthesis *Or* TORP, bypassing malleus
Absent	Absent	Intact	PORP
Absent	Absent	Only footplate present	TORP
Present	Present	Intact but fixed	Stapedotomy

PORP: partial ossicular reconstruction prosthesis; TORP: total ossicular reconstruction prosthesis.

6 Stapedotomy

SURGICAL STEPS

1 **Positioning the patient**
2 **Permeatal approach**
3 **Confirming the diagnosis and measuring**
4 **Dislocating the incudostapedial joint and removal of the stapes suprastructure**
5 **Fenestrating the stapes footplate**
6 **Positioning the prosthesis**
7 **Closure**

PROCEDURE

1 Positioning the patient

Position the patient on a head ring with the operating table head-up. Turn the patient's head away from the operative side. Prepare the skin with aqueous betadine solution to the ear and ear canal, and apply a head drape. Inject local anaesthetic in the form of 2% lignocaine with 1/80,000 adrenaline to the ear canal.

2 Permeatal approach

In the majority of cases, a permeatal approach allows adequate access; otherwise, consider an endaural incision.

Make a semicircular incision 10 mm from the annulus from 12 to 6 o'clock with a 45° round canal knife, raising a tympanomeatal flap with the drum elevator. Fold the flap forwards to expose the middle ear cavity. A fine curette may be needed to remove the bone overlying the stapes. The chorda tympani nerve should be preserved if possible; occasionally it may be necessary to sacrifice it for access. ✪

3 Confirming the diagnosis and measuring

Use a slightly curved needle to palpate the ossicular chain and confirm stapes fixation. Gently touch the malleus handle and observe reduced movement of the incus and fixation of the stapes. Measurement of the distance from the footplate to the lenticular process of the incus is made using the measuring rod (approximately 4.5 mm).

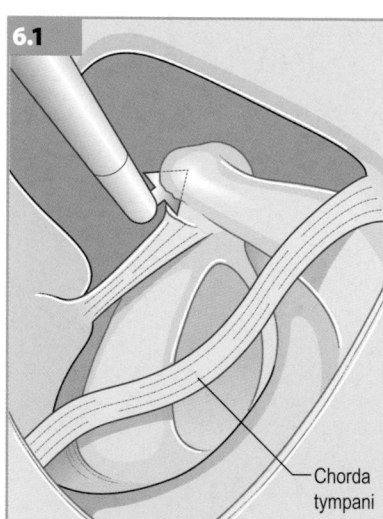

6.1 *The incudostapedial joint is separated with a joint knife.*

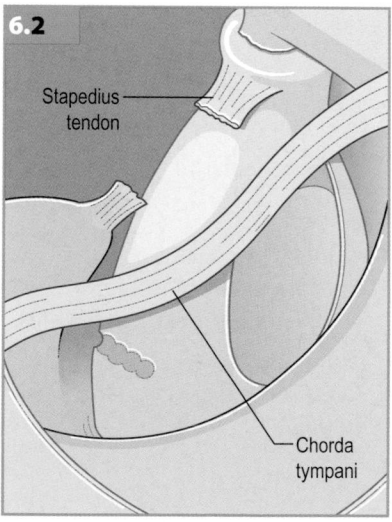

6.2 *Posterior crurotomy with KTP laser (incudostapedial joint and stapedius tendon are already divided).*

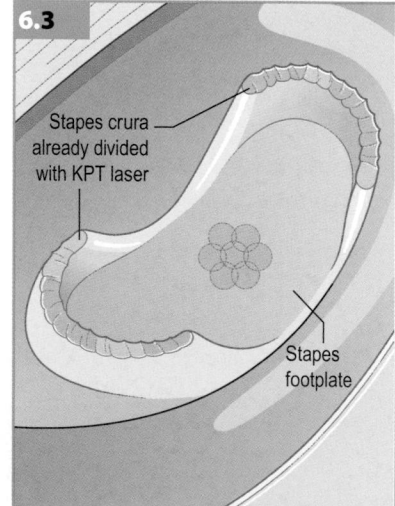

6.3 *Fenestration of the footplate.*

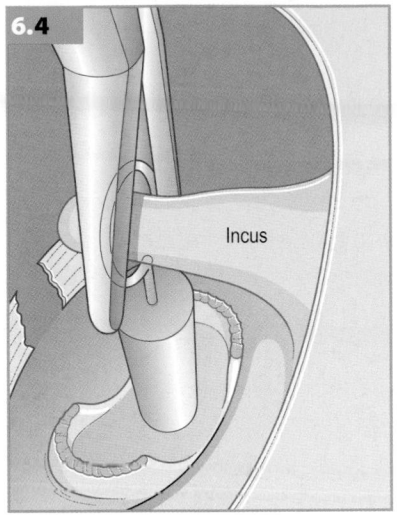

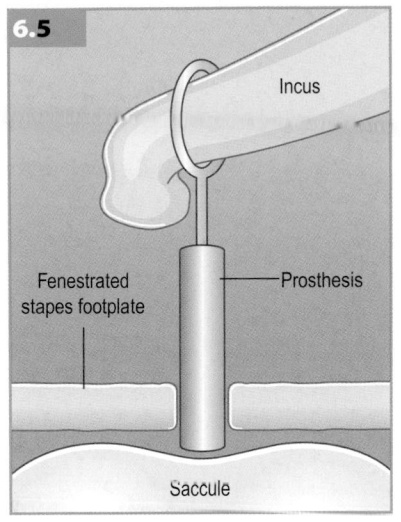

6.4 *Crimping the prosthesis.*

6.5 *Final positioning of prosthesis.*

☼ *Surgeon's tip* _____
*A standard aural speculum
can be fixed in place using a
transparent adhesive drape,
excising the drape over the
lumen.*

☼ *Surgeon's tip* _____
*Curetting should be directed
away from the ossicles to
prevent accidental damage.*

4 Dislocating the incudostapedial joint (ISJ) and removal of the stapes superstructure

The ISJ is disarticulated using the joint knife (**6.1**), and the stapedial tendon is cut from the posterior crus with microscissors. Using the right-angled pick or KTP laser, the crura of the stapes are fractured and the suprastructure is removed with cup forceps (**6.2**). ☼☼

5 Fenestrating the stapes footplate

Fenestration of the footplate is performed with a Skeeter drill (0.6 mm diamond burr) or KTP laser. Use irrigation to prevent excessive heating of the Skeeter drill. Complete the final part of the fenestration using a 0.6 mm trephine. Fenestration should be in the posterior half of the footplate; this avoids the prosthesis contacting the saccule (**6.3**).

6 Positioning the prosthesis

Select the appropriate prosthesis and trim If necessary to match the measurement. Crocodile forceps are used to place the prosthesis carefully into the fenestra and to crimp the free end around the lenticular process of the incus (**6.4**). Check final positioning of the prosthesis by palpating the ossicular chain (**6.5**). A fat plug may be placed around the stapedotomy site.

7 Closure

Replace tympanomeatal flap. In the ear canal put either a small pack or just Tri-AdCortyl ointment.

☼☼ *Surgeon's tip* _____
*A KTP laser can be used to divide
the stapes tendon, posterior
crus of stapes, and to perform
fenestration (with rosette
technique), as well as to crimp
the hook of some prostheses
(e.g. SMart prosthesis).*

7 Mastoidectomy and canalplasty

SURGICAL STEPS

1 **Positioning the patient**
2 **Examination under the microscope**
3 **Elevating the tympanomeatal flap**
4 **Surgical approaches:**
  – Postauricular
  – Endaural
5 **Harvesting the temporalis fascia graft**
6 **Cortical mastoidectomy**
7 **Canalplasty**
8 **Posterior tympanotomy**
9 **Positioning the graft**
10 **Packing and closure**

PROCEDURE

1 Positioning the patient

Position the patient on a head ring with the operating table head-up. Turn the patient's head away from the operative side. Attach a facial nerve monitor and ensure it is working (**7.1**). Shave the hair over the incision site. Inject approximately 10 ml of local anaesthetic and adrenaline in the form of 0.5% lignocaine and 1/200,000 adrenaline. Prepare the skin with betadine, and drape the patient tightly with a head drape to hold the hair out of the operative field.

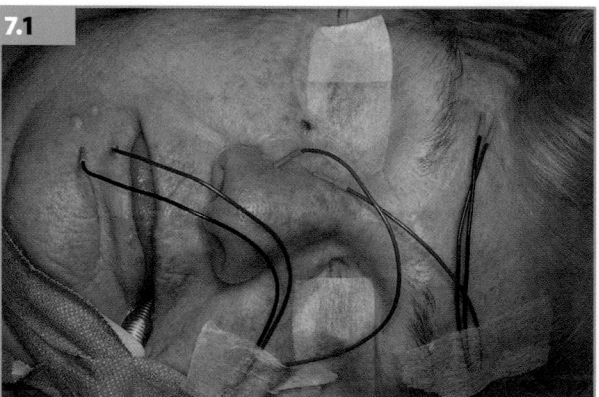

7.1 Facial nerve monitor on right side.

2 Examination under the microscope

Using the microscope, clean the ear canal and assess for perforation, attic defect, retraction pocket, and extent of cholesteatoma. Inject 1–2 ml of local anaesthetic in the form of 2% lignocaine with 1/80,000 adrenaline using a dental syringe. Inject slowly at the edge of hair-bearing skin from 12 o'clock to 6 o'clock. ✪

3 Elevating the tympanomeatal flap

Using a 45° round canal knife, make incision 5–10 mm lateral to the annulus, extending from 12 o'clock to 6 o'clock. Use a Plester D-knife to make two longitudinal incisions. Use the round canal knife to elevate the tympanomeatal flap until the annulus is reached or the cholesteatoma sac encountered. ✪✪

Lift the annulus out of the annular rim using a flat canal elevator to enter the middle ear space. ✪✪✪

Elevate the annulus from 12 o'clock to 6 o'clock. Use a curved needle to assess the continuity of the ossicular chain. If the ossicular chain is intact, moving the malleus will cause movement of the long process of the incus as well as the stapes suprastructure. In order to remove disease involving the ossicular chain, dislocate the long process of incus from the stapes suprastructure. In most cases the long process of the incus will have already been eroded by disease.

✪ *Surgeon's tip* _____
*The clock face used to describe the positions of the tympanic membrane or ear canal as shown in Figure **4.1**.*

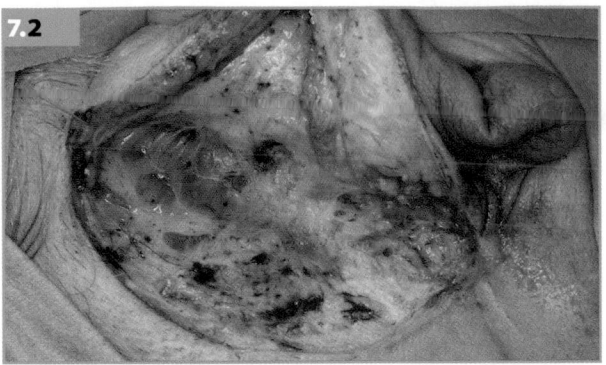

Surgeon's tip ⭐⭐

To avoid damage, do not allow the suction tip to touch the tympanomeatal flap. Always suction onto an instrument, or through cotton wool.

Surgeon's tip ⭐⭐⭐

To avoid damage to the ossicular chain and chorda tympani, start elevating the annulus in the postero-inferior quadrant.

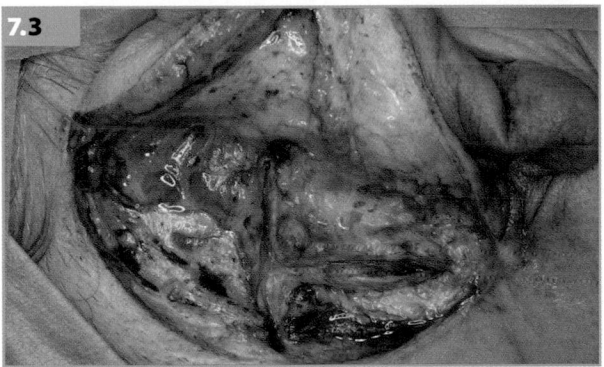

Surgeon's tip ⭐⭐⭐⭐

Holding the pinna between thumb and index finger, with the index finger in the external auditory meatus, retract the pinna anteriorly. Using a knife at 45° to the skull, dissect anteriorly in this plane, as far as the posterior edge of bony external auditory canal. This avoids damaging temporalis fascia or perforating the posterior external auditory canal skin.

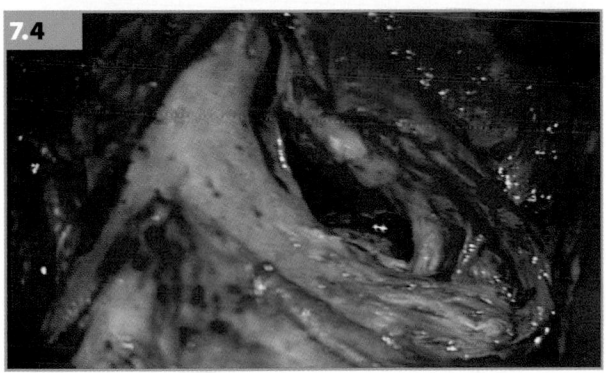

7.2–7.4 *Postauricular approach mastoidectomy.*

4 Surgical approaches
Postauricular

Using a 10 blade, make a skin incision 0.5–1 cm behind the postauricular sulcus, from the inferior margin of the external auditory meatus inferiorly to the level of the zygomatic arch superiorly (as in **4.2**). Continue the incision through the post-auricular muscles to the level of the temporalis fascia superiorly. Dissect as far as the posterior edge of bony external auditory canal (**7.2**). ⭐⭐⭐⭐

Using a 15 blade, make a T-shaped incision (**7.3**). Elevate the periosteum with a Freer elevator, taking care not to tear the periosteum or external auditory canal skin, especially at the spine of Henle. Enter the ear canal lumen using an incision through external auditory canal skin (**7.4**). Quarter-inch ribbon gauze is passed through the incision and the two ends held in a clip, retracting skin and pinna anteriorly. Insert two self-retaining retractors.

✪ Surgeon's tip
You can extend the superior end of the incision beyond the zygomatic arch, if needed.

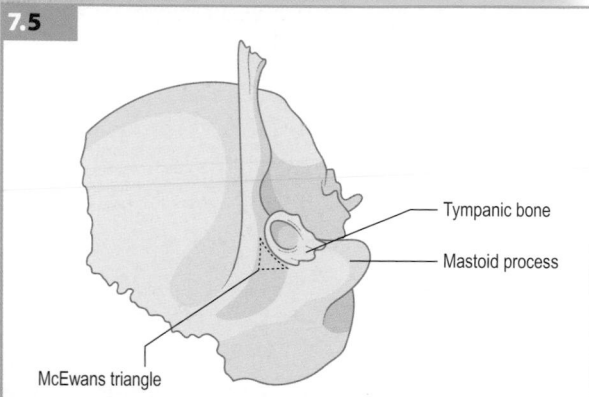

7.5 *Cortical mastoidectomy.*

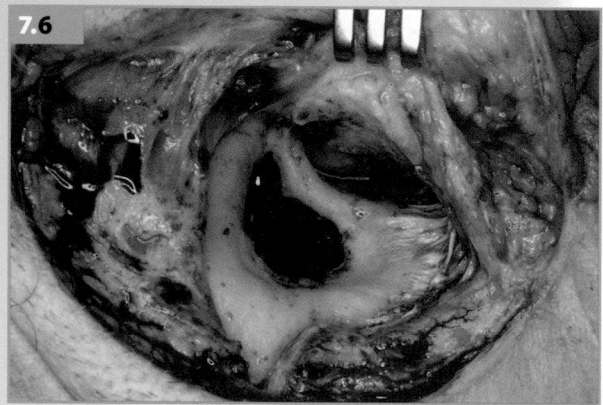

7.6 *Intraoperative photograph showing McEwan's triangle dissected.*

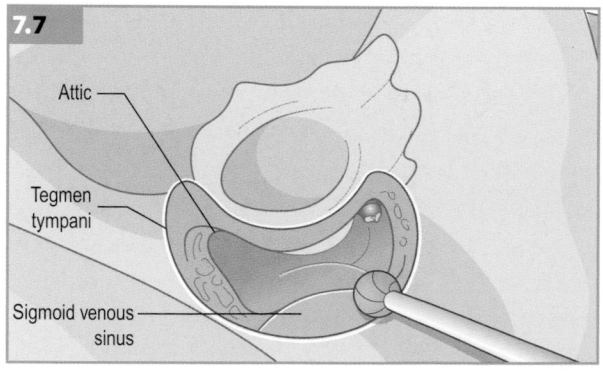

7.7 *Mastoid cavity*

Endaural
Using a 15 blade, make a skin incision between tragus and root of helix, and extend superiorly over the zygomatic arch as far as the temporalis fascia (as in **4.6**). Take care to avoid damaging cartilage. Using a Lempert speculum, extend the incision deep through the periosteum from the level of the zygomatic arch superiorly into the roof of the ear canal for 5 mm. Insert two self-retaining retractors. ✪

5 Harvesting the temporalis fascia graft
Lift the scalp with a Langenbeck retractor. Dissect plane above the temporalis fascia using scissors. Incise temporalis fascia, and separate fascia off muscle with a Freer elevator. Use nontoothed forceps and curved iris scissors to harvest the graft (size appropriate to the tympanic defect). Spread the graft out on a glass slide to dry.

6 Cortical mastoidectomy
Using a large cutting burr (size 6), mark the cortical mastoidectomy bony edges using as landmarks the root of the zygomatic arch and the spine of Henle, creating an inverted triangle down to the tip of the mastoid (**7.5, 7.6**). First remove the cortical bone before changing to a smaller burr (size 4) to remove the honeycomb structure of the mastoid cavity. Expose the tegmen tympani (cortical bone of the anterior cranial fossa floor).

Thin the bone over the lateral venous sinus, again using the drill parallel to the cortical bone. Drill antero-superiorly to expose the attic (**7.7**). Thin down the posterior bony canal wall, taking great care to avoid drilling through the cortical bone of the lateral semicircular canal. Having exposed the attic, identify the body of the incus. You have successfully completed the cortical mastoidectomy. ✪✪

7 Canalplasty

If the external auditory canal is very narrow or tortuous, a canalplasty may be required to provide access to the whole of the middle ear cavity and annulus. Bony spicules can be individually removed to improve access, but often a more thorough canalplasty is required. Use a Plester D-Knife to make longitudinal incisions in the external auditory canal skin at 12 o'clock and 6 o'clock, running laterally from the tympanomeatal flap to the junction of the bony and cartilaginous external auditory canal. Retract the flaps laterally and secure them under the self retainer, or insert a temporary stay suture.

Once the bone has been exposed, use a cutting burr size 2 or 3, to widen the external auditory canal. In order to avoid inadvertently opening the glenoid fossa and temporomandibular joint, remove bone anterosuperiorly and anteroinferiorly first, in a 'kidney-bean' shape. Then carefully drill the bridge of bone left between the two, making sure to leave a thin layer of bone over the fibres of the temporomandibular joint.

8 Posterior tympanotomy

Using a small (size 2) cutting burr carefully thin the posterior canal wall. Use the lateral semicircular canal and the body of the incus as landmarks (**7.8**). Start close to the incus and move inferiorly. The width of dissection is approximately 1 mm and the length 2–3 mm. When the bone is thinned adequately, the middle ear cavity can be entered medial to the annulus, at the level of the facial recess. You have successfully completed the posterior tympanotomy. All disease can now be removed. ✪✪✪

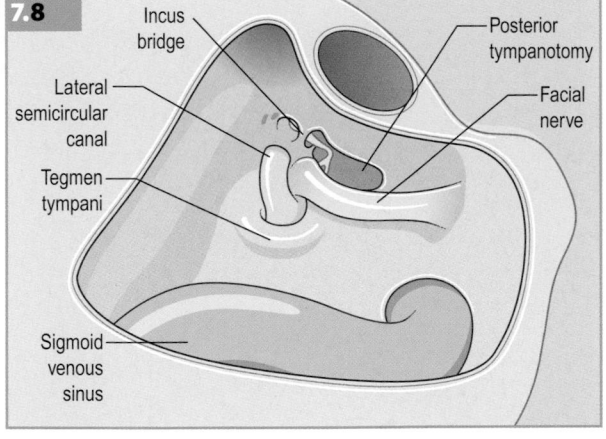

7.8 *Right posterior tympanotomy*

Incus bridge
Posterior tympanotomy
Lateral semicircular canal
Facial nerve
Tegmen tympani
Sigmoid venous sinus

✪✪ Surgeon's tip
To avoid perforating the tegmen, use the drill in a parallel direction to the cortical bone. Occasionally dura may be exposed, but as long as it is not breached, no further action is required.

✪✪✪ Surgeon's tip
On completion of the posterior tympanotomy, a 30° rigid scope can be inserted to assess for any residual disease.

✪ *Surgeon's tip* _____

Management of mastoiditis complicated by a subperiosteal abscess may require emergency insertion of a grommet and drainage of the abscess. Use the skin incision described above and cautiously perform a cortical mastoidectomy; the procedure is completed when the pus is released.

✪ *Surgeon's tip* _____

If a canalplasty has been performed, the ear canal pack may need to be replaced for a further 2–3 weeks at the first postoperative appointment, to prevent stenosis of the external auditory canal.

9 Positioning the graft

Cut the graft to size. Holding the front edge of the graft in a pair of crocodile forceps, place underneath the tympanic membrane, ensuring the graft covers the defect. Place some pieces of sofradex-soaked absorbable gelatin sponge in the middle ear to support the graft. Replace the tympanomeatal flaps.

10 Packing and closure

Pack the deep ear canal with pieces of absorbable gelatin sponge and/or bismuth iodoform paraffin paste (BIPP). Mastoidectomy incisions are closed with 3/0 vicryl to periosteum and 4/0 prolene to skin. A pressure bandage of paraffin impregnated gauze such as Jelonet®, gauze, cotton wool, and crepe bandage is applied overnight. ✪

8 Cochlear implantation

SURGICAL STEPS

1 **Positioning the patient**
2 **Postauricular incision**
3 **Cortical mastoidectomy**
4 **Posterior tympanotomy**
5 **Package bed**
6 **Cochleostomy**
7 **Implant insertion (+/– testing)**
8 **Closure**

PROCEDURE

1 Positioning the patient

Position the operating table head-up. Turn the patient's head away from the operative side. Attach a facial nerve monitor and ensure it is working (as shown in **7.1**). Shave hair over the incision site. Inject approximately 10 ml of local anaesthetic and adrenaline in the form of 0.5% lignocaine and 1/200,000 adrenaline. Prepare the skin with betadine, and drape the patient tightly with a head drape to hold the hair out of the operative field. Use opsite dressing to hold the pinna anteriorly, sealing the external auditory canal from the surgical incision site. ✪

2 Postauricular incision

Using a 10 blade, make a skin incision in the postauricular sulcus, from the inferior margin of the external auditory meatus inferiorly and then extending vertically upwards into the scalp, to just past the tip of the pinna (**8.1**). Continue the incision through the postauricular muscles to the depth of the periosteum inferiorly, and to the level of the temporalis fascia superiorly. Using a 15 blade, make a parallel incision in the periosteum, 1 cm posterior to the skin incision. Elevate the periosteum anteriorly with a Freer elevator, taking care not to tear the periosteum or external auditory canal skin, especially at the spine of Henle. Expose the external auditory canal roof.

3 Cortical mastoidectomy

Using a large cutting burr (size 6), mark the cortical mastoidectomy bony edges using as landmarks the root of the zygomatic arch and the spine of Henle, creating an inverted triangle down to the tip of the mastoid (*see* **7.5**, **7.6**). First remove the cortical bone before changing to a smaller burr (size 4) to remove the honeycomb structure of the mastoid cavity. Expose the tegmen tympani (cortical bone of the anterior cranial fossa floor).

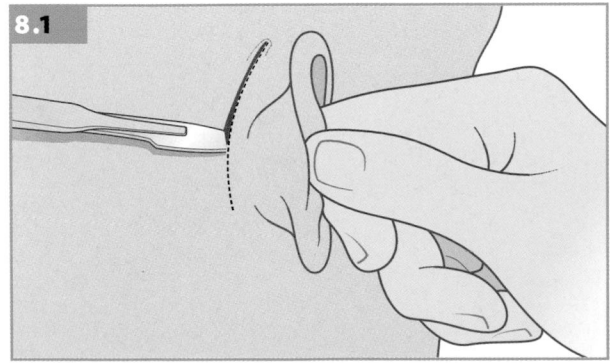

8.1

8.1 *Postauricular incision.*

✪ **Surgeon's tip** ───────────
To minimise the risk of infection, use the double glove technique to prepare and drape the patient, then discard the outer pair of gloves.

✪ **Surgeon's tip** _____
To avoid perforating the tegmen, use the drill in a parallel direction to the cortical bone. Occasionally the dura may be exposed, but as long as it is not breached, no further action is required.

✪✪ **Surgeon's tip** _____
Try not to breach the inner table of bone of the skull when drilling the package bed. In young children with very thin skulls, this may be impossible to avoid, in which case protect the underlying dura with a Freer's sucker as you drill.

✪✪ **Surgeon's tip** _____
Some implants no longer require a package bed to be drilled, and the implant can be positioned directly underneath the periosteum.

Drill antero-superiorly to expose the attic (*see* **7.8**). Thin down the posterior bony canal wall, taking great care to avoid drilling through the cortical bone of the lateral semicircular canal. Having exposed the attic, identify the body of the incus. The cortical mastoidectomy for a cochlear implant can be less extensive than in middle ear disease cases, as long as the lateral semicircular canal and short process of incus are identified. ✪

4 Posterior tympanotomy

Leaving a small bony incus bridge, drill the posterior tympanotomy with a 1.5 curved cutting burr (if available), or 2 mm then 1 mm standard straight burr. Start close to the incus and move inferiorly. The width of dissection is approximately 1 mm and the length 2–3 mm. When the bone is thinned adequately the middle ear cavity can be entered medial to the annulus. Saucerise the posterior tympanotomy to provide as much space as possible as shown in Figure **8.2**.

5 Package bed

Use a Freer elevator to create a periosteal pocket for the processor. The pocket should be at 45° posterosuperior to the external auditory canal (**8.3**). Drill the package bed with a size 4 mm cutting burr, and use a 2 mm cutting burr to make a channel leading from the package bed to the cortical mastoidectomy. Some surgeons drill two suture holes to secure the package in place. ✪✪

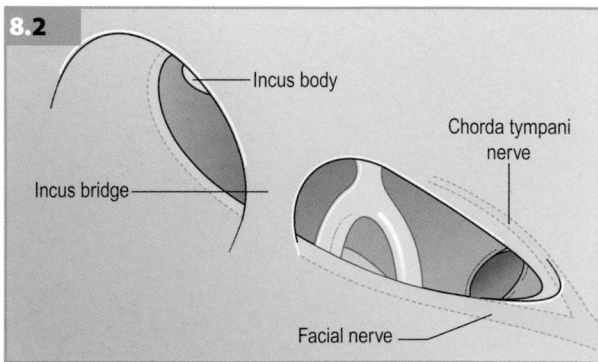

8.2 *Posterior tympanotomy.*

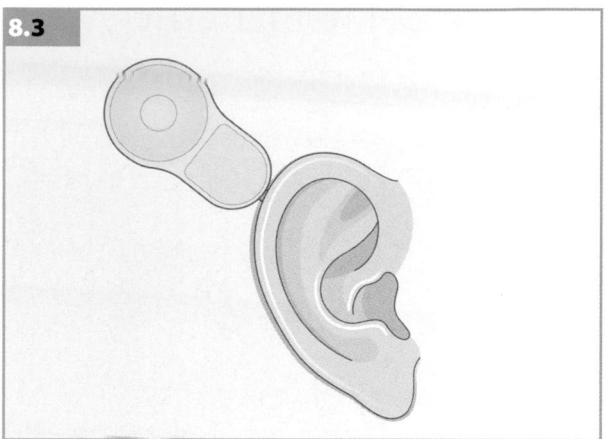

8.3 Package bed.

7 Implant insertion (+/– testing)

Change your gloves to minimise any risk of device infection. Position the processor under the temporalis fascia in the bony well (if drilled). Incise the cochlear endosteum. Insert the electrode using the insertion device as far as marker point. Use fascia or muscle to plug the cochleostomy around the implant. Anchor the electrode wires at the posterior tympanotomy and mastoid cortex using bone wax.

8 Closure

Closure is in layers with 3/0 vicryl and 4/0 monocryl, followed by steri-strips. Perform neural response testing if required. Apply a head bandage.

6 Cochleostomy

Using a 1 mm curved diamond drill, perform the cochleostomy via the posterior tympanotomy. The cochleostomy should be performed anteroinferior to the round window (**8.4**). Continue drilling until the white colour of the endosteum is visualised. Try to leave the endosteum intact to minimise trauma to the cochlea – the 'soft surgery' technique.

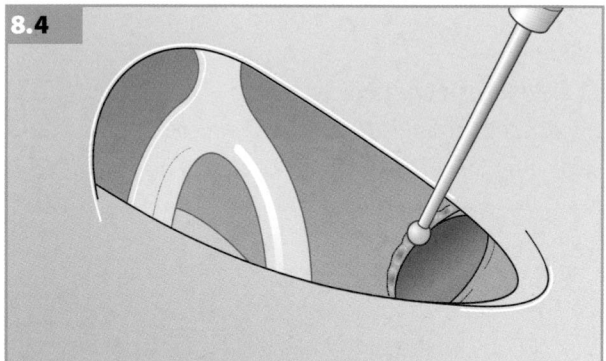

8.4 Cochleostomy.

9 Manipulation under anaesthesia of fractured nose (Closed reduction of acute nasal fracture)

SURGICAL STEPS

1. **Assessing the deformity**
2. **Disimpacting and reducing the nasal bone fracture**
3. **Manipulating the septum if required**
4. **Dressing and packing if required**

PROCEDURE

1 Assessing the deformity
Assess the deformity by standing at the head of the bed and looking down the nasal bridge. Nasal anatomy is shown in Figure **9.1**.

2 Disimpacting and reducing the nasal bone fracture
Disimpact nasal bones by first pressing on the side of the depressed nasal bone. Place the balls of both thumbs at the base of the nasal bone and press medially. Once bones are mobile, manipulate them to midline, and close any open roof deformity (**9.2**). Use Walsham forceps to lift out nasal bones, if they have collapsed medially. Rubber tips on the external forcep protects the facial skin.

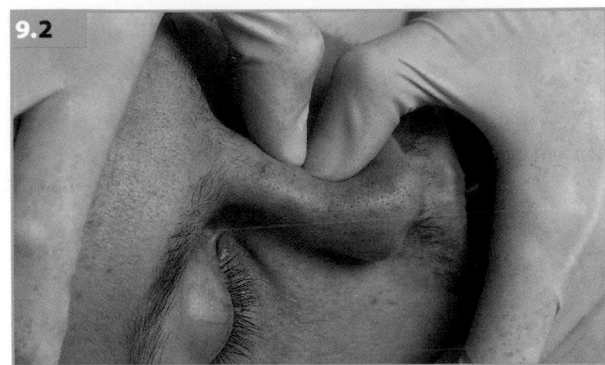

9.2 *Disimpacting the nasal bone fracture.*

3 Manipulating the septum if required
Use Asch forceps to manipulate minor septal deviations. Perform septoplasty in severe septal deviations (*see 10 – Septoplasty*). ✪

4 Dressing and packing if required
Insert intranasal packs to support excessively mobile nasal bones. Use elastoplast tape to skin over the nasal dorsum, or plaster-of-Paris if nasal bones are very mobile.

✪ **Surgeon's tip** _____
Unless septal deviation is very severe, it is better to wait a few months until all oedema has resolved.

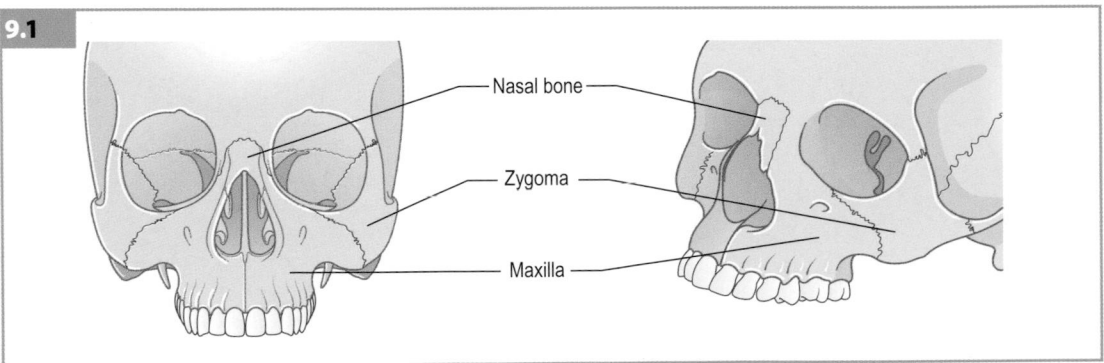

9.1 *Nasal bone anatomy.*

10 Septoplasty

SURGICAL STEPS

1 **Positioning the patient**
2 **Assessing the deformity and tip support**
3 **Incision and raising mucoperichondrial flaps**
4 **Mobilising the quadrilateral cartilage**
5 **Excising the perpendicular plate of ethmoid and vomerine spurs**
6 **Correcting the cartilaginous deformity**
7 **Excising maxillary crest spurs**
8 **Packing and closure**

PROCEDURE

1 Positioning the patient

Moffatt's solution, or an alternative, is applied in both nasal fossae of the anaesthetised patient 10 minutes prior to the procedure. Drape the patient with a head drape. Position the operating table head-up (**10.1**).

2 Assessing the deformity and tip support

Using a Killian's speculum, assess the septal deformity. Check that the nasal tip is adequately supported, and palpate the septum to confirm whether the quadrilateral cartilage is intact.

Inject local anaesthetic in the form of 2% lignocaine with 1/80,000 adrenaline using a dental syringe to the anterior 1/3 of the septum; usually 2–3 cartridges are necessary. Inject in the subperichondrial plane to achieve bloodless dissection. ✪

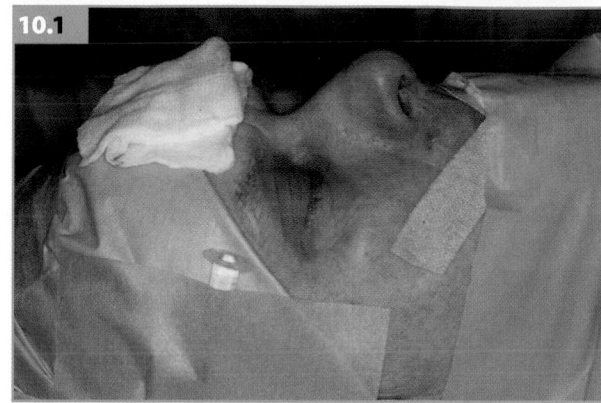

10.1 *Positioning the patient.*

> ✪ **Surgeon's tip**
> *Deformity is frequently due to excess cartilage anteriorly which must be excised, while maintaining tip support.*

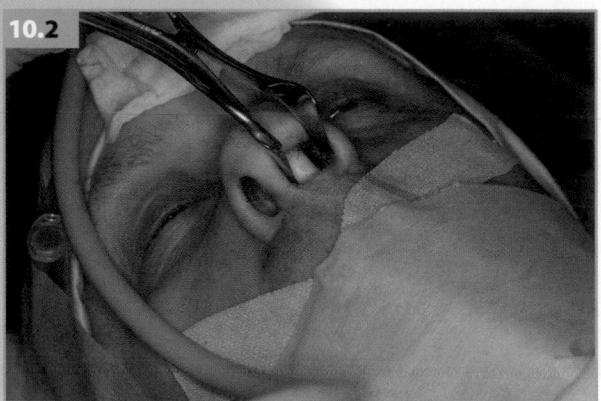

10.2 *Site of left hemitransfixation incision.*

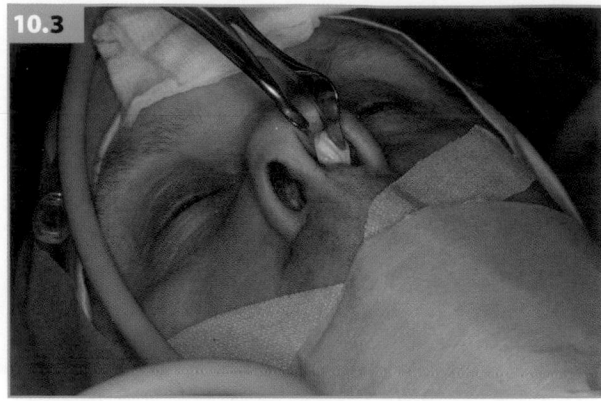

10.3 *Anterior edge of quadrilateral cartilage exposed.*

3 Incision and raising mucoperichondrial flaps

It is the senior author's practice always to perform a left hemitransfixion incision. Use a Killian's speculum to stabilise vestibular skin and septal mucosa (**10.2**). Using a 15 blade, make a vertical incision through the mucosa and perichondrium down to cartilage. This hemitransfixion incision should be along the anterior edge of the quadrilateral cartilage, i.e. the leading edge (**10.3**).

A shiny, bluish tinge characterises the cartilage, and shows that the subperichondrial plane has been reached. Using a Killian's speculum and Freer elevator, elevate the left mucoperichondrial flap as far as the osseocartilaginous junction, with the perpendicular plate of ethmoid posteriorly. ✪

Continue the dissection inferiorly onto vomer. Then dissect anteriorly, along the inferior border of the quadrilateral cartilage, working from posterior to anterior. Ensure that the maxillary crest is fully exposed (**10.4** shows septal anatomy).

4 Mobilising the quadrilateral cartilage

Using a Freer elevator, dislocate the quadrilateral cartilage from the perpendicular plate of ethmoid and vomer posteriorly. Dislocate the quadrilateral cartilage from the maxillary crest inferiorly, using either a Freer elevator or hockey stick, leaving the anterior strut attached to the maxillary spine if possible to provide tip support.

5 Excising the perpendicular plate of ethmoid and vomerine spurs

With a Freer elevator, raise the mucoperiosteal flap posteriorly bilaterally and remove the anterior strip of bone to enable the cartilage to move freely. Resect any bony spurs causing functional obstruction using punch forceps, e.g. Jansen–Middleton forceps. ✪✪

✪ Surgeon's tip

It is easier to elevate the mucoperichondrial flap superiorly, as it is less adherent to cartilage here.

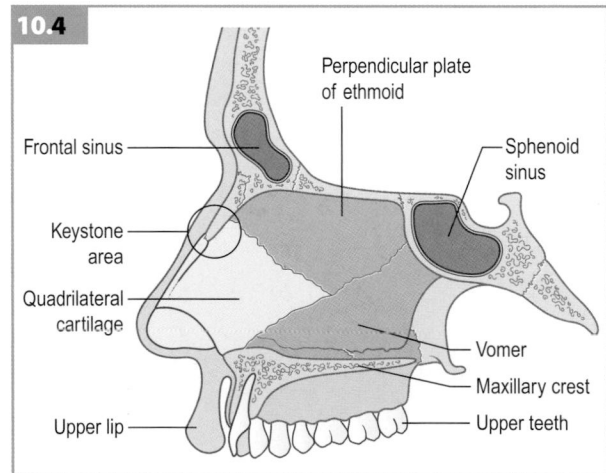

10.4 *Septal anatomy.*

6 Correcting the cartilaginous deformity

Deliver the anterior edge of the quadrilateral cartilage through the hemitransfixion incision and, if the cartilage is deviated secondary to excess height, excise an inferior strip of quadrilateral cartilage with a 15 blade. Take care not to reduce the height of the quadrilateral cartilage anteriorly, otherwise tip support will be compromised. Excise any fracture lines (**10.5**). ✪✪✪

7 Excising maxillary crest spurs

Use hammer and fishtail gouge to remove maxillary crest spurs (**10.6**).

8 Packing and closure

Reassess the septum and ensure there is no residual deformity. Check mucoperichondrial flaps are intact and that tip support is adequate. If the quadrilateral cartilage has been detached from the maxillary spine, use a 4/0 PDS suture to reattach the cartilage to the anterior nasal spine. Pass the needle through the quadrilateral cartilage and mucosa bilaterally, then pick up the periosteum of the maxillary crest on ipsilateral and then contralateral side, and tie.

Close the incision with 4/0 vicryl rapide, and use a quilting suture to minimise risk of postoperative haematoma.

The senior author does not routinely use nasal packs, but if excessive bleeding has been encountered packing will minimise the risk of postoperative haematoma.

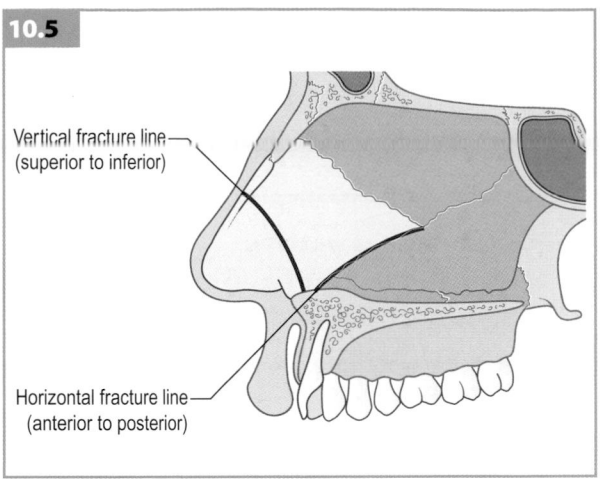

Vertical fracture line (superior to inferior)

Horizontal fracture line (anterior to posterior)

10.5 *Fracture lines in septum.*

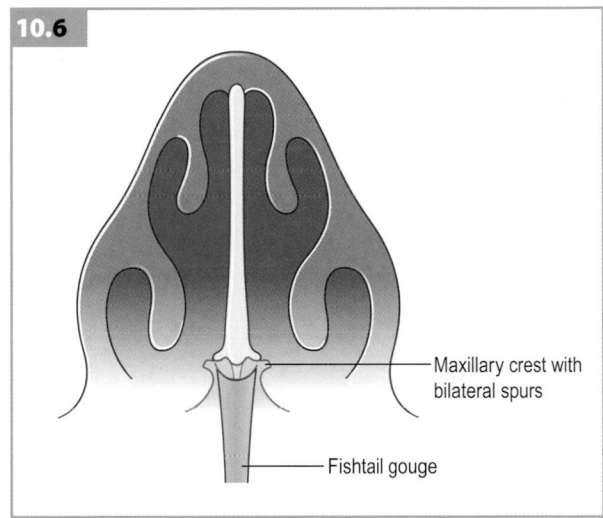

Maxillary crest with bilateral spurs

Fishtail gouge

10.6 *Excision of maxillary crest spur with fishtail gouge.*

✪✪ Surgeon's tip _____

Take care to leave the keystone area intact, where the osseo-cartilaginous junction joins nasal bones.

✪✪✪ Surgeon's tip _____

Scoring the concave surface of the quadrilateral cartilage can improve minor deflections. Use a 15 blade to incise serially the perichondrium.

11 Surgery to inferior turbinates

SURGICAL STEPS

1 **Positioning the patient**
2 **Examination of the nasal cavities**
3a **Submucosal diathermy**
3b **Linear diathermy**
3c **Outfracture**
3d **Turbinoplasty**

PROCEDURE

1 Positioning the patient

Moffatt's solution (*Table 11.1*), or an alternative, is applied in both nasal fossae of the anaesthetised patient 10 minutes prior to procedure. Drape the patient with a head drape and position the operating table head-up. ✪

2 Examination of the nasal cavities

Use a rigid nasendoscope to examine both nasal cavities.

3a Submucosal diathermy

Insert an Abbey monopolar diathermy needle submucosally along the length of the inferior turbinate, avoiding contact with the periosteum. Cauterise whilst slowly withdrawing the needle. Repeat the insertion and cautery two to three times (11.1, 11.2). ✪✪

3b Linear diathermy

Apply an Abbey monopolar diathermy needle along the surface of the inferior turbinate. Cauterise while slowly withdrawing the needle. Repeat cautery two to three times.

✪ Surgeon's tip

A number of alternative modalities are available, including laser ablation and radiofrequency treatment, but these are beyond the scope of this book.

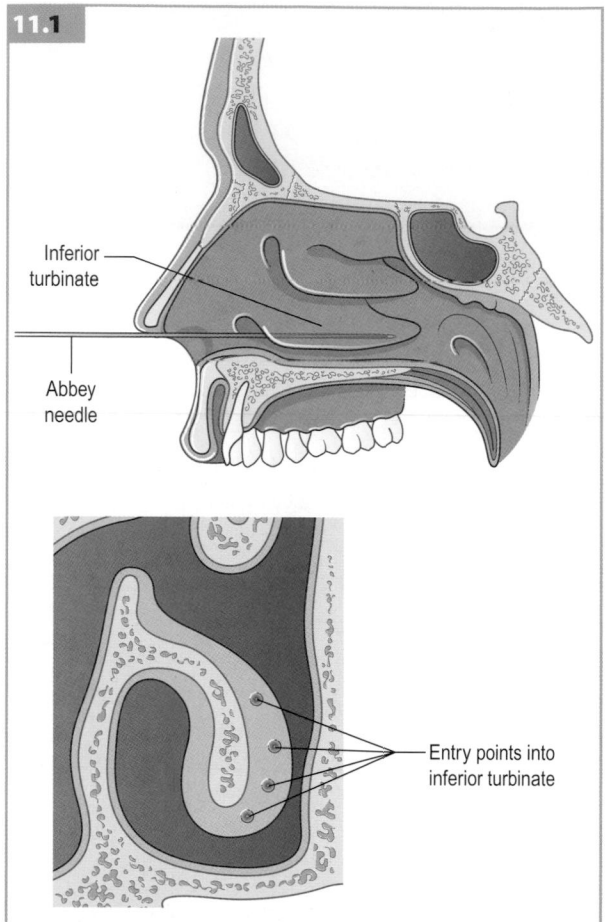

11.1 *Diagram showing insertion of an Abbey needle along the whole length of the inferior turbinate.*

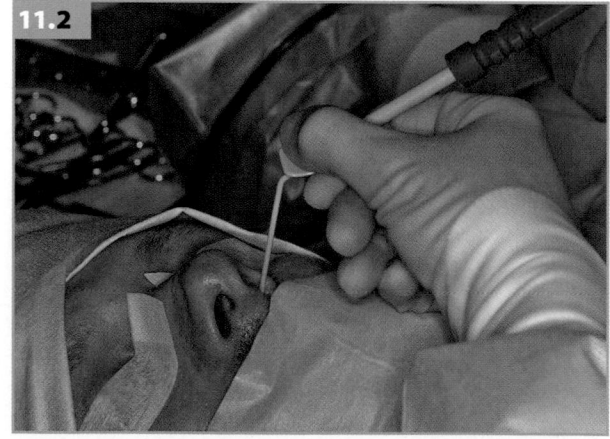

11.2 *Submucosal diathermy*

3c Outfracture

Using a Hills elevator, apply pressure to the lateral aspect of the anterior end of the inferior turbinate and medialise the turbinate. Repeat the procedure four to five times along the length of the turbinate. Once the turbinate has been mobilised, gently use a Hills elevator to lateralise it (**11.3, 11.4**). ✪✪✪

3d Turbinoplasty

Using a microdebrider or sickle knife, make an incision along the inferior border of the inferior turbinate. Use a Freer or a Cottle's elevator to elevate the mucoperiosteum off the bone of the turbinate, and remove the bone with a Blakesley forceps. Reapproximate the edges, and pack with an absorbable haemostatic sheet such as Surgicel® – this can be removed in the outpatient clinic in 1 week – or a dissolvable dressing.

✪✪ *Surgeon's tip*

In order to prevent thermal injury to skin or mucosa, avoid any contact between the diathermy tip and other surgical instruments, and always use an insulated nasal speculum.

✪✪✪ *Surgeon's tip*

Apply antibiotic nasal cream to the nasal cavities at the end of the procedure. Nasal packing is not routinely required.

Table 11.1: MOFFATT'S SOLUTION

Preparation	Comments
5 ml solution containing: • 1ml 1/1000 adrenaline • 2 ml 10% cocaine • 2 ml 8.4% sodium bicarbonate	• Moffatt's solution is usually prepared and instilled by the anaesthetist • Other alternatives may be considered as it has a potential toxicity, particularly for cardiac patients • Alternatives include Otrivine (xylomatazoline) or adrenaline

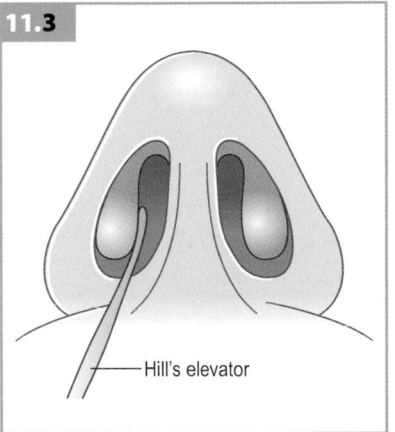

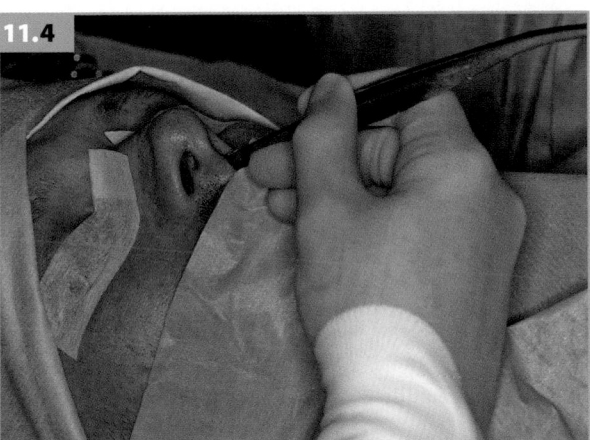

11.3, 11.4 *Outfracture of the inferior turbinate.*

12 Endoscopic sphenopalatine artery ligation

SURGICAL STEPS

1 **Positioning the patient**
2 **Identifying the sphenopalatine artery (SPA)**
3 **Ligating the SPA**

PROCEDURE

1 Positioning the patient

Moffatt's solution, or an alternative, is applied in both nasal fossae of the anaesthetised patient 10 minutes prior to the procedure. Drape the patient with a head drape, keeping the eyes exposed. Position the operating table head-up.

2 Identifying the SPA

Remove packs only when the patient is anaesthetised and you are ready to start the procedure with all equipment available. Examine the relevant nostril with a 4 mm, 0° rigid nasal endoscope. Infiltrate 1–2 ml of 2% lignocaine with adrenaline 1/80,000 in the region of the posterior insertion of the middle turbinate. Using a 15 blade, make a 1 cm vertical mucosal incision along the lateral nasal wall, 1 cm posterior to the middle meatus (**12.1**). ✪

Use a Freer elevator to elevate a mucosal flap of the lateral nasal wall as far as the crista ethmoidalis. Carefully continue elevation to expose the SPA and nerve. Curettage of crista ethmoidalis may be necessary.

3 Ligating the SPA

Ligate the SPA using vascular ligature clips (**12.2**). Endoscopic bipolar diathermy may also be used. Replace the mucoperiosteal flap. ✪✪

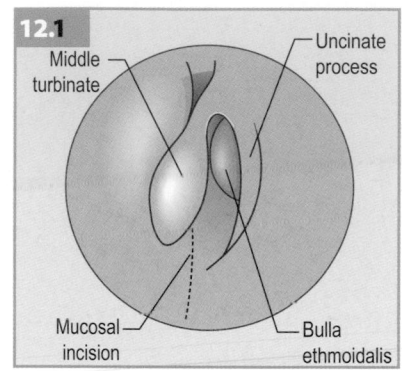

12.1 *The incision.*

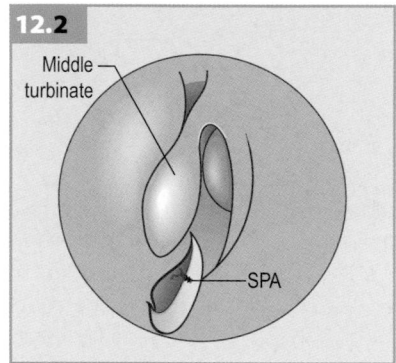

12.2 *Exposing the sphenopalatine artery (SPA).*

✪ **Surgeon's tip**
Some surgeons advocate making a small middle meatal antrostomy to aid correct placement of the incision.

✪✪ **Surgeon's tip**
It is possible to perform a maxillary artery ligation if SPA ligation fails. This is beyond the scope of this book, and many surgeons would advocate embolisation of the maxillary artery or ligation of the external carotid artery in an emergency situation (see 19 – External carotid artery ligation).

13 Anterior ethmoidal artery ligation

SURGICAL STEPS

1 **Positioning the patient**
2 **Marking and local anaesthetic**
3 **Dissecting and identifying the anterior ethmoidal artery (AEA)**
4 **Ligating the AEA**

PROCEDURE

1 Positioning the patient
Moffatt's solution, or an alternative, is applied in both nasal fossae of the anaesthetised patient 10 minutes prior to the procedure. Drape the patient with a head drape, keeping the eyes exposed. Position the operating table head-up.

2 Marking and local anaesthetic
Mark a 2–3 cm curved incision midway between the inner canthus and nasal bridge – the classical Lynch incison. Inject local anaesthetic in the form of 2% lignocaine with 1/80,000 adrenaline using a dental syringe (**13.1**). ✪

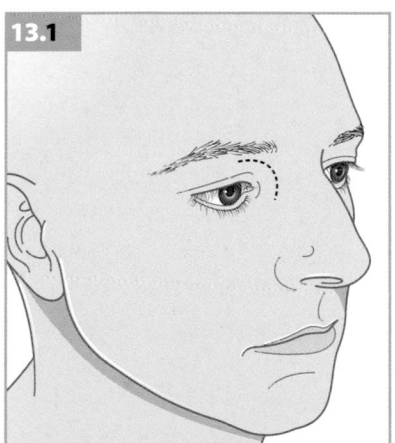

13.1 Marking a Lynch incision.

✪ **Surgeon's tip** _____
*Perform tarsorrhaphy to protect the eye (**13.2**, **13.3**).*

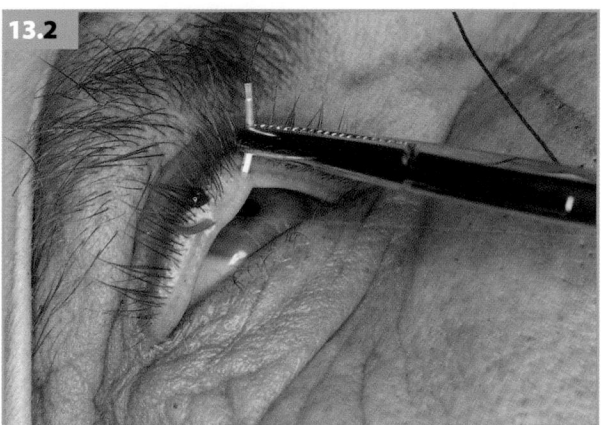
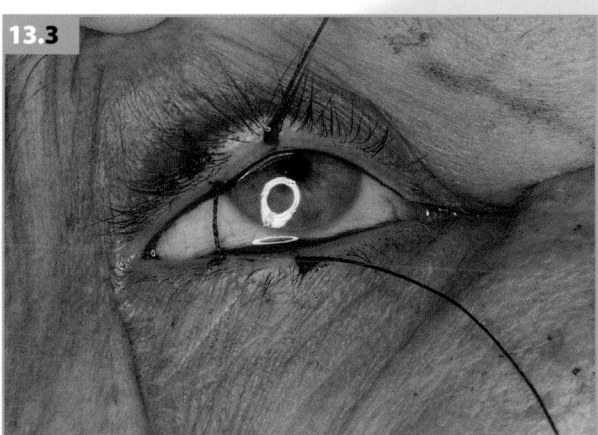

13.2, 13.3 Perform a tarsorrhaphy.

✪✪ *Surgeon's tip*

Mnemonic rule of 24–12–6 indicates the relation between anterior EA–posterior EA–optic nerve.

✪✪✪ *Surgeon's tip*

It is possible to perform a maxillary artery ligation if AEA ligation fails. This is beyond the scope of this book, and many surgeons would advocate embolisation of the maxillary artery or ligation of the external carotid artery in an emergency situation (see 19 – External carotid artery ligation).

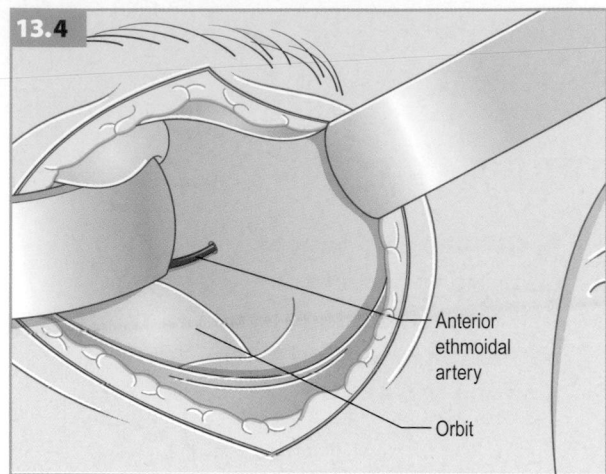

13.4 *Dissecting and identifying the anterior ethmoidal artery.*

3 Dissecting and identifying the AEA

Incise the skin down to the periosteum with a 15 blade. Use a Freer elevator to lift the periosteum laterally. Lateralise the lacrimal sac and expose the lacrimal bone and lamina papyracea. Use a malleable copper retractor to retract gently the periosteum and orbit contents laterally. Identify the AEA approximately 24 mm from the anterior lacrimal crest (**13.4**). ✪✪

4 Ligating the AEA

Ligate the AEA using vessel ligature clips. Also use bipolar diathermy at a low setting to avoid damage to the optic nerve. Use a small corrugated drain, and 6.0 prolene to close the wound. ✪✪✪

14 Functional endoscopic sinus surgery (FESS)

SURGICAL STEPS

1   **Positioning the patient**
2   **Septoplasty if required**
3   **Uncinectomy**
4   **Middle meatal antrostomy**
5   **Anterior ethmoidectomy**
6   **Posterior ethmoidectomy**
7   **Sphenoidotomy**
8   **Frontal recess**

PROCEDURE

1 Positioning the patient

Moffatt's solution, or an alternative, is applied in both nasal fossae of the anaesthetised patient 10 minutes prior to the procedure. Drape the patient with a head drape, keeping the eyes exposed. Position the operating table head-up. Attach a 4 mm 0° Hopkins rod to a light source, camera, and stack system. Focus the camera on the nasal tip, and white balance the image against a swab. Place a wet swab on the patient's forehead for cleaning the scope, and dip the tip of the scope in antifog solution. Apply two neuropatties with topical adrenaline, strength 1/1000 diluted with 5 ml normal saline in the middle meati bilaterally. Wait 2 minutes. ✪

2 Septoplasty if required

Septoplasty is completed if necessary for access to the middle meati (*see 10 – Septoplasty*).

3 Uncinectomy

Remove the neuropatties from the middle meatus. Medialise the middle turbinate gently using a Freer elevator. Identify the uncinate process by palpating the lateral nasal wall with the Freer until you feel the bone of the uncinate process give way. Use an angled Freer or sickle knife to make a single incision from superior to inferior, detaching the uncinate process from the lateral nasal wall. Use Mackay forceps to detach the uncinate process from the lateral wall of the nose superiorly. Using straight Blakesley forceps, remove the uncinate process in its entirety (mucosa and bone) to expose the infundibulum (**14.1**). Place adrenaline-soaked neuropatties in the middle meatus to control bleeding, and repeat on the contralateral side ✪✪

✪ *Surgeon's tip*
Before you begin, have the CT scans available in the operating theatre, and take care to review the scans systematically and thoroughly to avoid any surprises during the procedure.

✪✪ *Surgeon's tip*
Place all tissue removed from the nasal cavity in a gallipot. Any floating tissue may signify fat, and the operation should be paused while operative progress and exact positioning are carefully checked.

✪✪ *Surgeon's tip*
Use cutting forceps to detach the uncinate process from the lateral nasal wall, to avoid avulsing bone and mucosa, which might cause a CSF leak from the anterior cranial fossa.

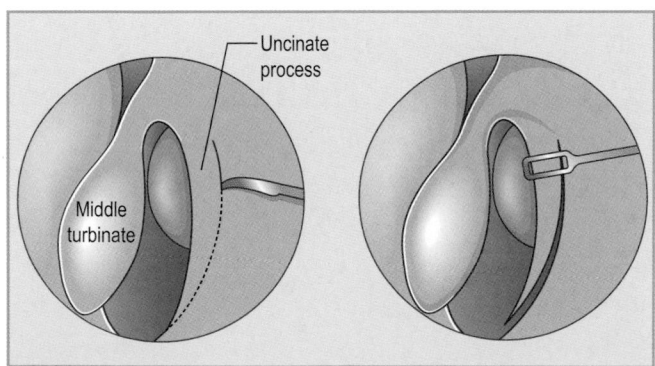

Uncinate process

Middle turbinate

14.1 *Uncinectomy.*

✪ *Surgeon's tip* _____
To avoid damage to the naso-lacrimal duct, do not cut through hard lacrimal bone when using the back-biting forceps.

✪ *Surgeon's tip* _____
Some surgeons advocate the Wigand or back to front technique. Identification of the MMA, followed by sphenoid sinus position, allow appreciation of the height of the skull base to aid safe posterior ethmoidectomy.

4 Middle meatal antrostomy

Widen the opening into the maxillary sinus, using backbiting through-cutting forceps to widen the antrostomy anteriorly, and Mackay through-cutting forceps to widen it posteriorly. ✪

5 Anterior ethmoidectomy

Identify ethmoid bulla and hiatus semilunaris (*see anatomy in* **14.2**). Perforate and open the anterior wall of bulla and open the anterior ethmoid air cells using a curette or straight Blakesley forceps, and clear all bony partitions to expose the skull base. Laterally, beware of breaching the lamina papyracea. If you are in doubt, ballot the ipsilateral eye, and confirm that there is no sign of any movement along the lateral wall.

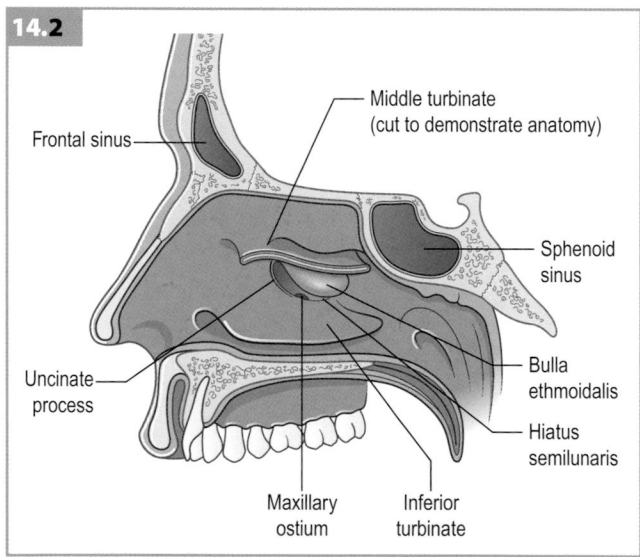

14.2 *Anatomy of ethmoid bulla and hiatus semilunaris.*

6 Posterior ethmoidectomy

If posterior ethmoidectomy is required, then approach this through the ground lamella. This is identified intraoperatively as a vertical sheet of bone at the junction of the anterior and posterior ethmoids. Using a curette or small sucker, perforate the ground lamella and confirm your position. You can now remove the remaining ground lamella and enter the posterior air cells and clear as necessary. Pack with adrenaline-soaked neuropatties, and repeat steps on the contralateral side.

7 Sphenoidotomy

Identify the posterior choana, and using a Ferguson sucker, walk up the posterior nasal wall, just medial to the midpoint of the choanal arch. After approximately 1 cm, you should identify the slit-like opening of the sphenoid ostium. Confirm your position by pushing the sucker tip through the ostium. Using a sphenoid punch, widen the ostium. Do not attempt to clear the contents of the sphenoid sinus without supervision, as the internal carotid artery and optic nerve lie in the lateral wall. ✪

8 Frontal recess

Frontal recess surgery is not part of a routine FESS operation, and as such should only be undertaken with appropriate training and supervision. ✪✪

✪ *Surgeon's tip* _____
When widening the sphenoid ostium, avoid straying too far inferiorly, where you may encounter the septal branch of the sphenopalatine artery.

✪✪ *Surgeon's tip* _____
Emergency sequelae of sinusitis such as orbital cellulitis with subperiosteal abscess, or orbital abscess, can also be treated endoscopically. Follow the steps as described, cautiously looking for the abscess cavity. It may be necessary to remove the lamina papyracea to release the pus. Use copious vasoconstrictors as the inflammation makes the procedure particularly difficult. If the abscess cannot be drained endoscopically it may be necessary to use a Lynch Howarth incision to drain the abscess via the external approach, as described in 13 – Anterior ethmoidal artery ligation.

✪✪ *Surgeon's tip* _____
In revision or complex cases, image guided navigation systems can provide invaluable real-time information, although obviously are no substitute for sound anatomical knowledge.

15 Septorhinoplasty

SURGICAL STEPS

1 **Positioning the patient**
2 **Septoplasty**
3 **Intercartilagenous incisions**
4 **External/open approach**
5 **Sub-superficial musculoaponeurotic system (SMAS) dissection**
6 **Dehumping**
7 **Medial osteotomies**
8 **Lateral external osteotomies and infracture of nasal bones**
9 **Suturing and plaster**

PROCEDURE

1 Positioning the patient

Moffatt's solution, or an alternative, is applied in both nasal fossae of the anaesthetised patient 10 minutes prior to the procedure. Drape the patient with a head drape, keeping the eyes exposed (**15.1**). Position the operating table head-up. Inject local anaesthetic in the form of 2% lignocaine with 1/80,000 adrenaline using a dental syringe; usually 4–5 cartridges are necessary. Inject local anaesthetic to:
- The anterior 1/3 of septum bilaterally.
- The intercartilagenous incision.
- The nasal hump.
- Nasal bones.

2 Septoplasty

Septoplasty is completed (*see 10 – Septoplasty*) using a left hemitransfixion incision.

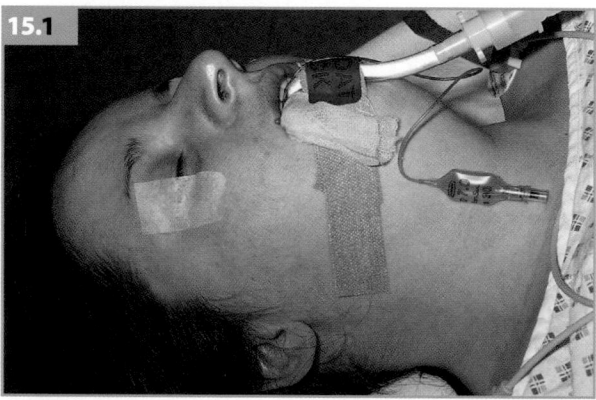

15.1 *Positioning the patient.*

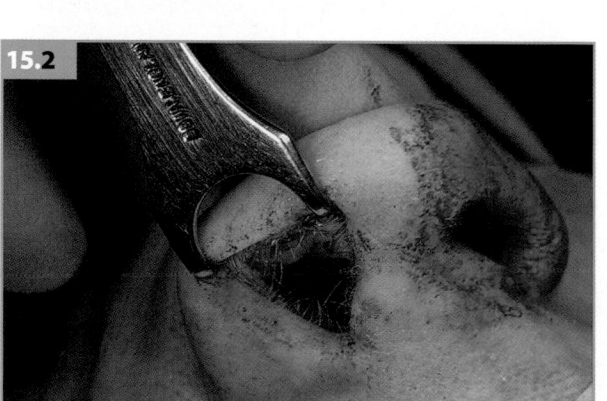

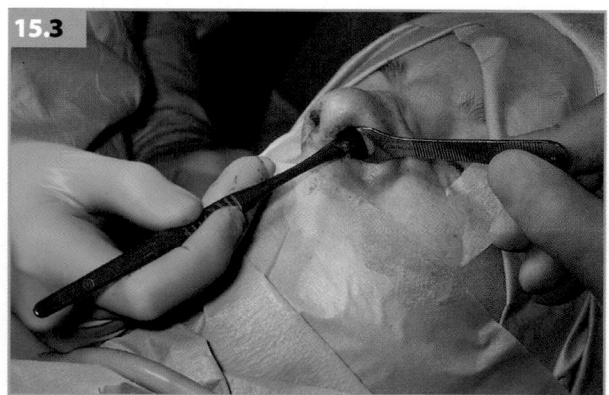

15.2, 15.3 *Intercartilaginous incisions.*

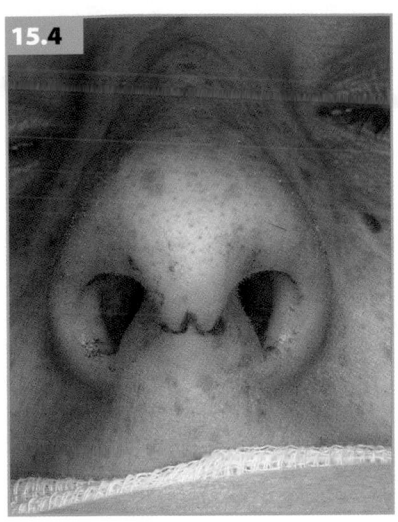
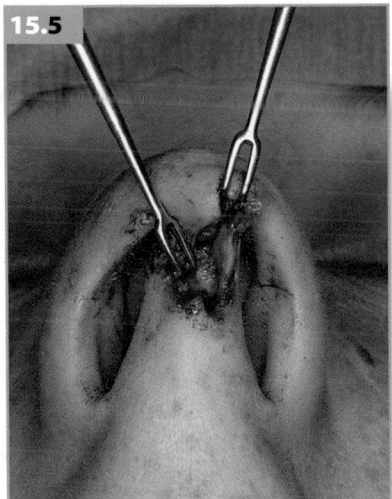
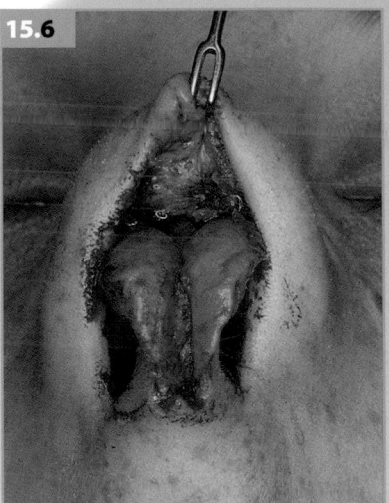

15.4–15.6 *External/open approach.*

3 Intercartilaginous incisions

Once septoplasty is completed, use an alar retractor to retract the alar rim (**15.2**) and a 15 blade to perform intercartilagenous incisions (**15.3**). The intercartilagenous incision should be connected to the hemitransfixion incision on the left side. On the right side, the incision should run along the septum down the superior 1/3 of the columella, posterior to the medial crura of the lower lateral cartilage.

4 External/open approach

Use an inverted V or W columella skin incision to expose the nose (**15.4**). Using the 15 blade cut through the columella skin, taking care to avoid damaging the medial crurae of the lower lateral cartilages. Expose the rest of the tip of the nose until you have completely exposed the lower lateral cartilages (**15.5**, **15.6**). ✪

5 Sub-SMAS dissection

Complete the sub-SMAS dissection using McIndoe scissors. Separate the bony and cartilaginous nasal bridge from the nasal skin dorsally. Laterally, dissect the skin from the nasal bones so the nasal hump is fully exposed. Complete the dissection by connecting intercartilagenous incisions anterior to the quadrilateral cartilage (**15.7**). ✪✪

✪ **Surgeon's tip** _____
Place your columella incision midway along the columella length to avoid postoperative scar contracture.

✪✪ **Surgeon's tip** _____
Sub-SMAS dissection can also be completed using a 15 blade. Place an index finger on the surface of the nasal bridge. Trace a gentle circular movement of the 15 blade to avoid perforating the skin of the nose.

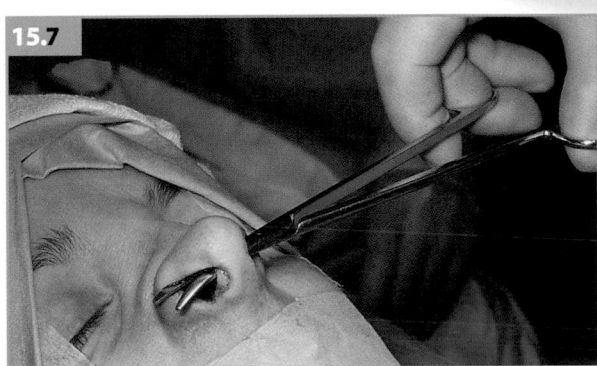

15.7 *Connecting intercartilagenous incision using McIndoe scissors.*

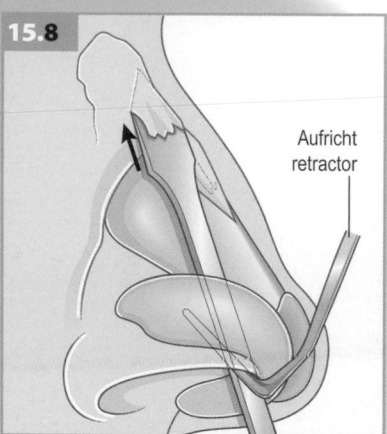

15.8 *Dehumping.*

⚙ Surgeon's tip ⎯⎯⎯⎯⎯⎯

It may be necessary to remove a further small amount of cartilagenous hump or part of the upper lateral cartilages. This can be done with a 15 blade under direct vision using an Aufricht retractor.

6 Dehumping

Use an Aufricht retractor to lift the skin of the nasal bridge and expose the cartilagenous and bony hump. Use a Howarth elevator to separate the procerus muscle from the upper part of the bony nasal hump. Assess the amount of bony and cartilagenous hump that needs to be excised. Use a 15 blade to incise the cartilagenous hump from anterior to posterior. Insert a flat, broad, 8 10 mm osteotome under the incised cartilagenous part of the hump, holding the osteotome in the right hand (**15.8**). Use the left index finger and thumb over the nasal skin to control the osteotome externally. Ask an assistant to tap, in a controlled manner, and stop when the osteotome has reached the superior limit of bony hump. Insert an Aufricht retractor and visualise the osteotomised hump. Use forceps to remove the hump under direct vision. Assess the cosmetic result externally; if necessary use nasal bone raspers to smooth the edge of nasal bones. ⚙

7 Medial osteotomies

Insert a 6–8 mm flat osteotome into the nasal fossa, parallel to the septum, and engage the blade at the anterior edge of the nasal bone, in the midline. Use the fingers of the left hand to guide the tip of the osteotome under the skin. Ask an assistant to tap until just before the blade reaches the glabellar cortical bone. Curve the blade laterally in the final few millimetres, so that the fracture line will meet subsequent lateral osteotomies (**15.9**).

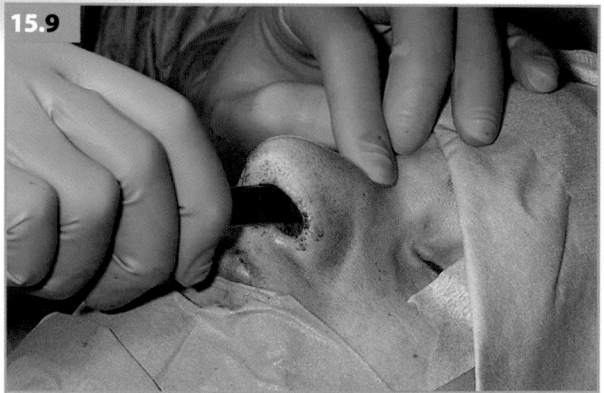

15.9 *Medial osteotomies.*

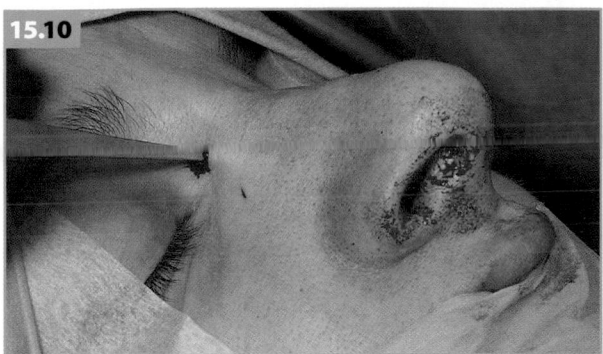

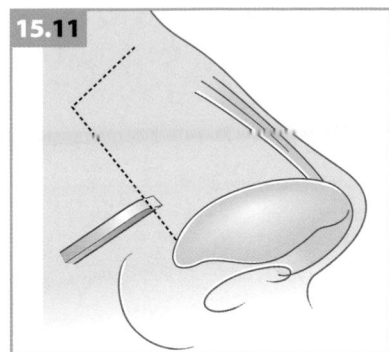

15.10, 15.11 *Lateral external osteotomies and infracture of nasal bones.*

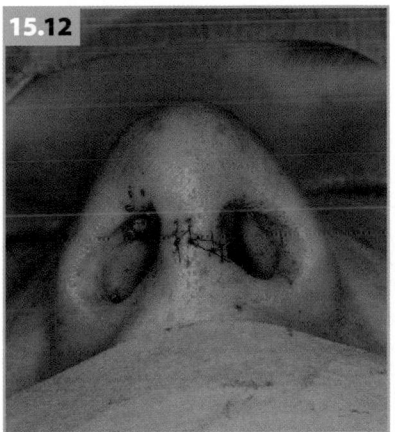

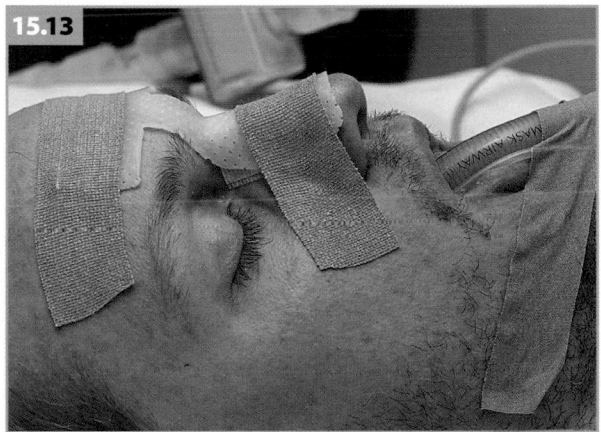

15.12 *Suturing.*

15.13 *Thermoplasty.*

8 Lateral external osteotomies and infracture of nasal bones

Use a 15 blade to make two stab incisions through the skin of the lateral wall of the nose, following natural skin creases (**15.10**), and use a swab to apply pressure to avoid bruising. Use a 2 mm osteotome to osteotomise the nasal bone bilaterally (**15.11**). Use a wet swab to perform infracture of nasal bones in a controlled manner. Assess the cosmetic result.

9 Suturing and plaster

Use undyed 4/0 vicryl to close septal and intercartilagenous incisions. Use 5/0 or 6/0 ethilon for the columella incision (**15.12**). Cover the skin of the nose with ½ inch steri-strips and apply a plaster-of-Paris splint (or thermoplasty as shown in **15.13**). ✪✪

✪✪ *Surgeon's tip* _____
The author advocates the use of 16 mg intravenous dexamethasone just before the end of the procedure to limit postoperative oedema.

16 Lateral rhinotomy and medial maxillectomy

SURGICAL STEPS

1 **Positioning the patient**
2 **Lateral rhinotomy incision**
3 **Exposure of the bony framework:**
   – Division of the trochlea
   – Exposure of the lacrimal sac
   – Exposure and mobilisation of the nasolacrimal duct
   – Division of anterior and posterior ethmoidal artery
   – Exposure of the infraorbital nerve
   – Elevation of the periosteum and nasal mucosa from the pyriform aperture
4 **Osteotomies – removal of specimen**
5 **Haemostasis and closure**

PROCEDURE

1 Positioning the patient

Moffatt's solution, or an alternative, is applied in both nasal fossae of the anaesthetised patient 10 minutes prior to the procedure. Mark the skin incision and infiltrate with local anaesthetic in the form of 2% lignocaine with 1/80,000 adrenaline solution (**16.1**). Position the patient on a head ring on the operating table. Position the operating table head-up. Drape the patient with a head drape, leaving the eyes exposed and prepare the skin with betadine. Using 4/0 prolene, secure the upper and lower lid of the eye on the operative side by performing a tarsorrhaphy (**16.2**, **16.3**). ✪

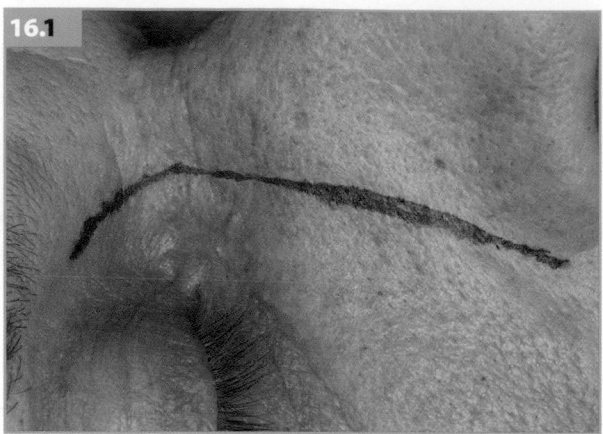

16.1 *Marking the site.*

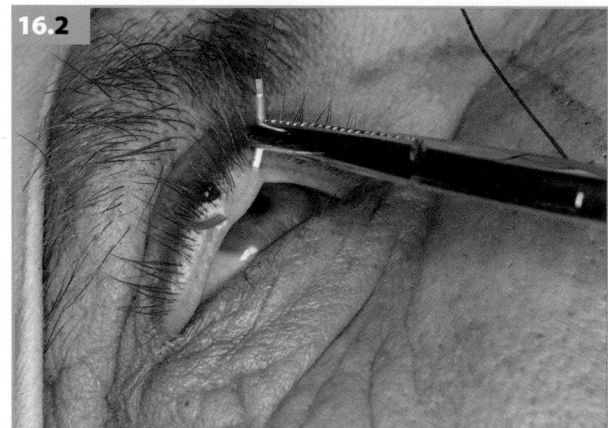

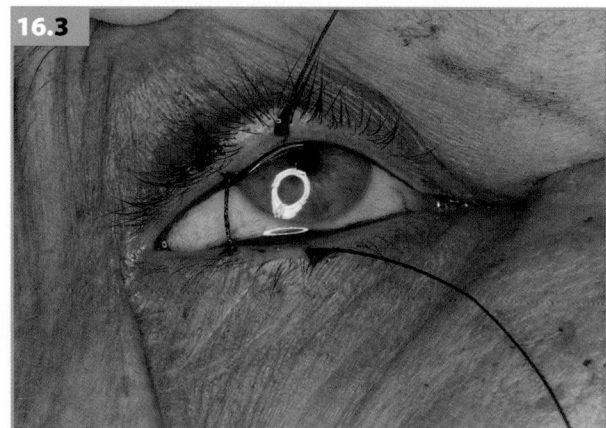

16.2, 16.3 *Perform a tarsorrhaphy.*

2 Lateral rhinotomy incision

Make an incision using a 15 blade, starting in the midpoint between the inner canthus and the nasal dorsum, proceeding inferiorly along the nasolabial line and curving around the alar rim as far as the mucocutaneous junction (**16.4**). ✪✪

3 Exposure of the bony framework

Using a Freer elevator, the periosteum is elevated from the maxillary bone, for 1 cm lateral to the nasomaxillary suture. ✪✪✪

Division of the trochlea

Elevate the periosteum of the medial orbital wall, and divide the trochlea as close as possible to the bone.

Exposure of the lacrimal sac

Continue dissecting medially and mobilise the lacrimal sac from the medial orbital wall, taking care not to damage the sac and duct.

Exposure and mobilisation of the nasolacrimal duct

Inferiorly the nasolacrimal duct inserts in the nasolacrimal bony canal. Remove maxillary bone from the inferior part of the bony canal using a Kerrison punch. Mobilise and divide the proximal part of the nasolacrimal duct. Enter the maxillary sinus and visualise the posterior and lateral walls to assess the extent of disease (**16.5**).

✪ *Surgeon's tip*

The senior author advocates the use of 16 mg dexamethasone at the beginning of the procedure.

✪✪ *Surgeon's tip*

Use bipolar diathermy as well as ribbon gauze soaked in 1/1000 adrenaline for haemostasis.

✪✪✪ *Surgeon's tip*

Care should be taken to avoid elevating the periosteum too far laterally and damaging the infraorbital nerve.

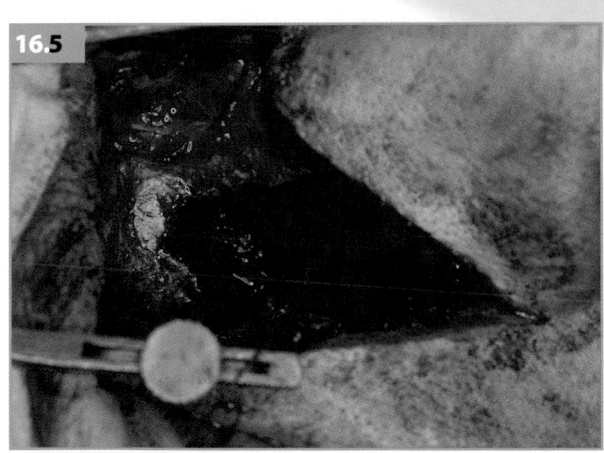

16.4 *Lateral rhinotomy incision.*

16.5 *Exposure and mobilisation of the nasolacrimal duct.*

Division of anterior and posterior ethmoidal artery

Dissect medially along the frontoethmoid suture for approximately 24 mm from the anterior lacrimal crest, and identify the anterior ethmoidal artery. Clip, ligate, or diathermy this vessel. If the tumour extends more posteriorly, continue dissecting a further 12 mm and ligate the posterior ethmoidal artery. ✪

Exposure of the infraorbital nerve

On the anterior wall of the maxilla, dissect laterally as far as the infraorbital nerve, as it emerges under the inferior orbital rim, taking care not to injure the nerve.

Elevation of the periosteum and nasal mucosa from the pyriform aperture

At the rim of the pyriform aperture, elevate the mucoperiosteum medially, exposing the medial wall of the pyriform aperture.

4 Osteotomies – removal of a specimen

Resection is tailored to the size and extension of the tumour. The limits of the resection are:

- Superiorly – just below the skull base (identified by the frontoethmoid suture line on the medial orbital wall).
- Inferiorly – floor of the maxillary sinus, including the inferior turbinate.
- Laterally – infraorbital nerve.

Strong curved Mayo scissors are used for cutting through the inferior anterior wall of the maxilla, while an osteotome can be used to remove the more superior lateral parts of the bony wall.

5 Haemostasis and closure

Feed a silastic O'Donoghue stent through the upper and lower lacrimal punctae, and advance it into the nasolacrimal duct. Anchor the trochlea and inner canthal ligament to the periosteum using 3/0 vicryl sutures. Closure is performed in two layers, using 3/0 vicryl for the subcutaneous tissues and periosteum and 5/0 prolene for the skin of the face. Pack the maxillectomy cavity with Whitehead's varnish ribbon gauze. ✪✪

✪ Surgeon's tip

Care must be taken with dissection, as the optic nerve lies just 4–6 mm posterior to the posterior ethmoidal artery.

✪✪ Surgeon's tip

Medial maxillectomy can also be performed endoscopically; however, specialist training is advocated before embarking on this.

17 Maxillectomy

SURGICAL STEPS

1. **Positioning the patient**
2. **Tarsorrhaphy**
3. **Weber Fergusson incision:**
   - Skin incision
   - Intraoral incision
   - Skin flap elevation
4. **Osteotomies**
5. **Packing and closure**

PROCEDURE

1 Positioning the patient

Position the operating table head-up. Place a head ring and sand bag under the patient's shoulder. Inject approximately 10 ml of local anaesthetic in the form of 0.5% lignocaine and 1/200,000 adrenaline. Prepare the skin with betadine, and drape the patient with a head drape.

2 Tarsorrhaphy

Using 4/0 prolene, secure the upper and lower lid of the eye on the operative side by performing a tarsorrhaphy (*see 16 – Lateral rhinotomy and medial maxillectomy, 16.2, 16.3*). ✪

3 Weber Fergusson incision
Skin incision

Using a 15 blade, make an incision midway between the medial canthus and the top of the nasal bridge. Extend the incision laterally along the lower eyelid as far as the lateral canthus. The incision runs 2–3 mm below the level of the eyelash. Inferiorly, continue the incision along the side of the nose into the alar groove and medially as far as the midline. Divide the upper lip up to the vermillion border. To avoid unsightly scarring, curve the incision as it runs through the lip (**17.1**).

Intraoral incision

Intraorally, the incision divides into two parts, gingivobuccal and palatal. Using cutting diathermy, continue the gingivobuccal incision laterally along the gingivobuccal sulcus as far as the maxillary tuberosity. The palatal part of the incision extends between the incisor teeth in the midline, to the hard palate until the junction of the hard and soft palate where it turns laterally behind the maxillary tuberosity to meet the gingivobuccal incision (**17.2**).

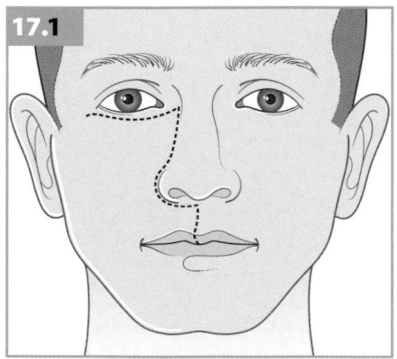

17.1 *Weber Fergusson skin incision.*

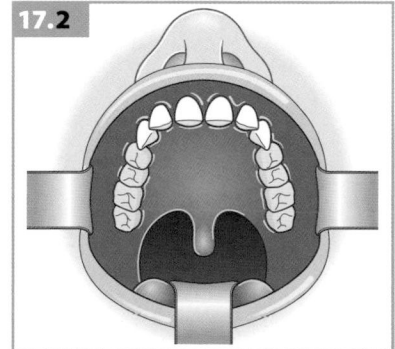

17.2 *Weber Fergusson intraoral incision.*

> ✪ **Surgeon's tip**
> *Make sure your tarsorrhaphy is made on the tarsal plate of the upper and lower lid and not on the mucosal surface of the lid to avoid the feeling of 'foreign body' following the operation. Also remember to remove the stitch after the procedure.*

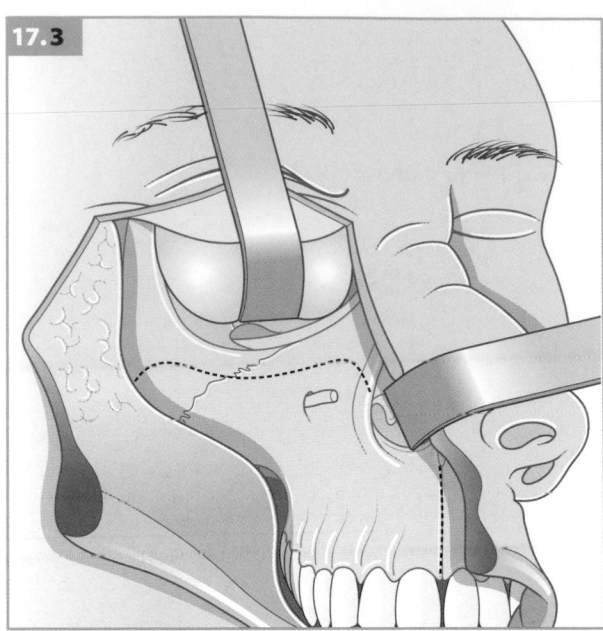

17.3 *Osteotomies on the surface of the maxilla.*

Skin flap elevation

Elevate the skin of the face over the maxillary bone using a periosteal elevator. Divide the infraorbital nerve and vessels. Extend the dissection to the level of the zygomatic arch. ✪

4 Osteotomies

Use a 2 mm drill burr to mark position of osteotomies on the surface of the maxilla (**17.3**). Starting laterally, the osteotomies extend from the zygomatic arch, below the infraorbital ridge, across the floor of the orbit to join the piriform aperture. The osteotomies continue inferiorly down the medial wall of the maxilla, detaching the middle turbinate and dividing the hard palate. Complete the osteotomies using an oscillating saw. Insert a curved osteotome behind the maxillary tuberosity and gently tap with a hammer whilst levering the maxilla forward, to detach it from the pterygoid plate. ✪✪

Once the maxilla has been mobilised, complete the dissection with McIndoe scissors to divide the pterygoid muscles and any soft tissue.

5 Packing and closure

Prior to the operation, a temporary dental plate with prosthesis is made which is then inserted at the end of the procedure to obturate the defect. Use 4/0 vicryl and 5/0 prolene to close the skin. Drainage is not necessary.

✪ **Surgeon's tip** _____

Skin flap elevation can also be carried out via a midfacial degloving approach, as described in 20 – Midfacial degloving.

✪✪ **Surgeon's tip** _____

Take care not to allow your osteotome to damage the contents of the pterygoid fossa, especially the pterygoid venous plexus. If you encounter bleeding in the pterygoid fossa, insert a large adrenaline-soaked tonsil swab and wait until the bleeding has stopped.

18 Endoscopic dacryocystorhinostomy

SURGICAL STEPS

This procedure is usually performed jointly with Ophthalmology. It may be performed under general or local anaesthesia.

1   **Positioning the patient**
2   **Inserting a lacrimal light probe**
3   **Creating a mucosal flap and exposing the lacrimal sac**
4   **Retrieving the light probe and inserting a stent**

PROCEDURE

1 Positioning the patient

Moffatt's solution, or an alternative, is applied in both nasal fossae of the anaesthetised patient 10 minutes prior to the procedure. If being performed under local anaesthesia, local anaesthetic is instilled to the eye and nose. Drape the patient with a head drape, keeping the eyes exposed. Position the operating table head-up. Inject local anaesthetic to the lateral wall of nose at an area of 1 cm × 1 cm anterior to the axilla of the middle turbinate in the form of 2% lignocaine with 1/80,000 adrenaline.

2 Inserting a lacrimal light probe

Insert a light probe via either superior or inferior canaliculus to the common canaliculus then into the lacrimal sac. This is easier if you stretch the eyelid laterally and follow the tract in a horizontal direction until the probe hits bone, and then turn the probe vertically downwards.

3 Creating a mucosal flap and exposing the lacrimal sac

The flap extends approximately 1 cm superior to the attachment of the middle turbinate and ends at the mid level of the uncinate process (**18.1**). Using a Freer elevator, peel the lacrimal bone off the lacrimal sac just anterior to the middle meatus. Remove the thin lacrimal bone. Use a dacryocystorhinostomy diamond burr to drill the frontal process of the maxillary bone that lies medially to the anterior 2/3 of the sac. Use a keratome to incise the lacrimal sac, making anteriorly and posteriorly based mucosal flaps (**18.2**).

4 Retrieving the light probe and inserting a stent

Remove the light probe and thread the metal ends of O'Donoghue tubes though the duct, taking care not to create a false passage. Remove the metal stents and make multiple knots in the tubes while taking care to leave a loose loop to avoid discomfort around the canaliculi.

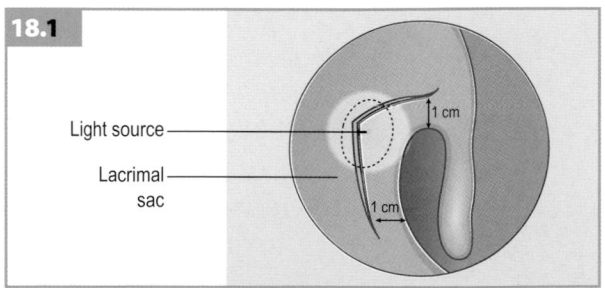

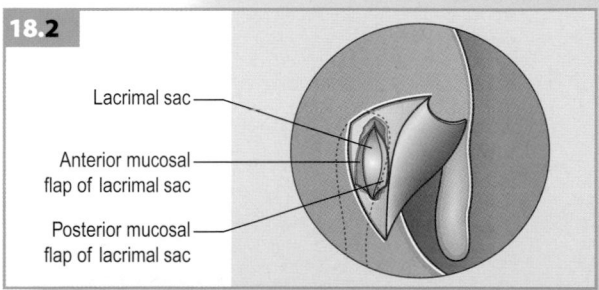

18.1, 18.2 *Mucosal flap.*

19 External carotid artery ligation

SURGICAL STEPS

1 **Positioning the patient**
2 **Incision and subplatysmal flaps**
3 **Identifying the carotid sheath**
4 **Identifying the external carotid artery**
5 **Haemostasis, drains, and closure**

PROCEDURE

1 Positioning the patient
Position the patient with a sandbag under the shoulders and head ring, and the operating table head-up. Use a marker pen to indicate the line of incision, 2–3 finger's breadth below the mandible in a skin crease and extending over the sternocleidomastoid muscle (**19.1**). Infiltrate with local anaesthetic in the form of 2% lignocaine and 1/200,000 adrenaline.

2 Incision and subplatysmal flaps
Using a 10 blade, incise through skin and platysma, preserving the great auricular nerve and external jugular vein in the posterior part of your incision. Ask your assistant to hold the skin flap under tension with catspaw retractors. Raise subplatysmal flaps, holding the blade parallel to platysma and staying directly on the under surface of the muscle to avoid damage to the marginal mandibular nerve, which will lie deep to the flap (*as in 35 – Neck dissection, 35.2*). Identify the anterior border of the sternocleidomastoid muscle.

3 Identifying the carotid sheath
Dissect along the anterior border of the sterno-cleidomastoid, while your assistant retracts the muscle posteriorly. Identify the carotid sheath, and then the common carotid artery. Put vascular slings around the common carotid for safety. ✪

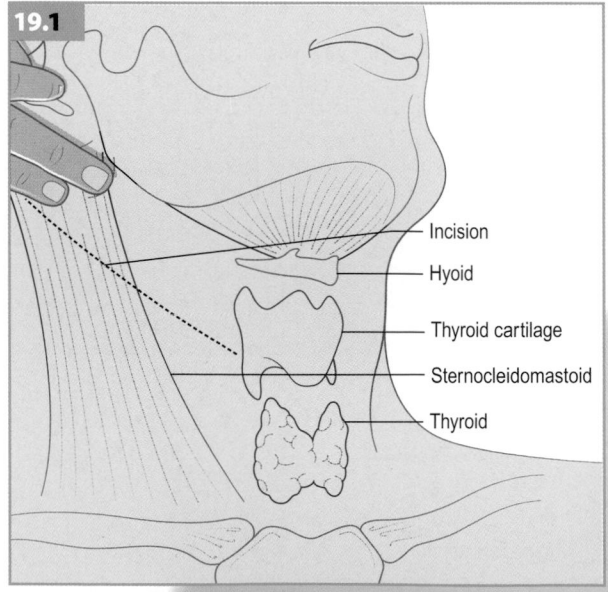

19.1

- Incision
- Hyoid
- Thyroid cartilage
- Sternocleidomastoid
- Thyroid

19.1 *Marking the incision.*

✪ Surgeon's tip
If bradycardia occurs when dissecting around the carotid bulb, inject 1% lignocaine with adrenaline into the vessel wall with a 23 gauge needle.

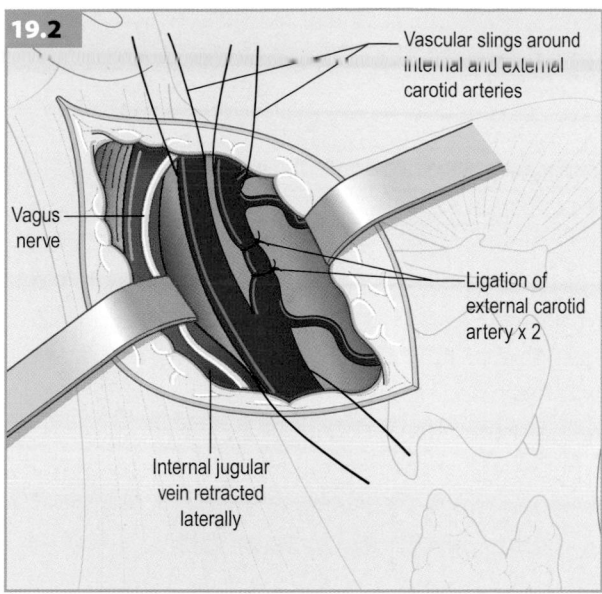

19.2

Vascular slings around internal and external carotid arteries

Vagus nerve

Ligation of external carotid artery x 2

Internal jugular vein retracted laterally

19.2 *Exposure of the external carotid artery*

4 Identifying the external carotid artery

Carefully dissect along the common carotid artery superiorly, towards the bifurcation, taking care not to damage the vessel. Look out for the hypoglossal nerve and avoid damaging it. Identify the carotid bifurcation, and subsequently the external carotid artery, which usually lies anterior and superficial to the internal carotid artery (**19.2**). You MUST identify the superior thyroid artery branching off the external carotid to be certain it is the correct vessel, and preferably the first two branches. Place two 0 silk ties around the external carotid artery, but do not divide the vessel.

5 Haemostasis, drains, and closure

Remove the vascular slings and ensure haemostasis; there is no need for a drain. Use 2/0 vicryl to close the platysma and deep subcutaneous layer. Apply skin staples and a transparent dressing such as Tegaderm®.

20 Midfacial degloving

SURGICAL STEPS

1 **Positioning the patient**
2 **Incisions – intraoral and intranasal**
3 **Exposure of the midface**
4 **Osteotomies and excision of the tumour**
5 **Closure**

PROCEDURE

1 Positioning the patient

Moffatt's solution is applied in both nasal fossae of the anaesthetised patient 10 minutes prior to the procedure. Drape the patient with a head drape, keeping the eyes and oral cavity exposed (*see* **15.1**). Position the operating table head-up. Inject local anaesthetic in the form of 2% lignocaine with 1/80,000 adrenaline using a dental syringe; usually 4–5 cartridges are necessary. Inject local anaesthetic to the:

- Anterior 1/3 of septum bilaterally.
- Intercartilagenous incision.
- Sublabial mucosa.

2 Incisions – intraoral and intranasal

Start with the intraoral incision. Using a 15 blade, incise sublabial mucosa down to the bone of the maxilla (**20.1**). Remember you can use the same incision for the Caldwell Luc approach to the maxillary sinus.

The intranasal incisions are as for a septorhinoplasty (*see 15 – Septorhinoplasty*). Perform a full transfixion incision, then use the alar retractor to retract the alar rim, and a 15 blade to perform intercartilagenous incisions. The intercartilagenous incision should be connected to the transfixion incision bilaterally. Continue the lateral end of the intercartilaginous incision to the floor of the nose and connect it with the transfixion incision behind the medial crura. ✪

3 Exposure of the midface

A periosteal elevator is used to elevate mucosa and skin from both sides of the maxilla and the intranasal and intraoral incisions are connected. Use McIndoe scissors to elevate the skin of the nose from the lower lateral and upper lateral cartilages, and nasal bones bilaterally. Use small Langenbeck retractors to retract the upper lip superiorly and use a periosteal elevator to separate the buccal mucosa from the anterior wall of the maxilla bilaterally as far as the infraorbital margin (**20.2**). ✪✪

4 Osteotomies and excision of the tumour

To expose the tumour, follow the principles of medial maxillectomy/lateral rhinotomy as described in *16 – Lateral rhinotomy and medial maxillectomy*. Excise the tumour, ensuring meticulous haemostasis and pack the nose and tumour cavity with a bismuth iodoform paraffin paste pack (BIPP).

5 Closure

Reposition the skin and use 4.0 vicryl to close both the intranasal and intraoral incisions. ✪✪✪

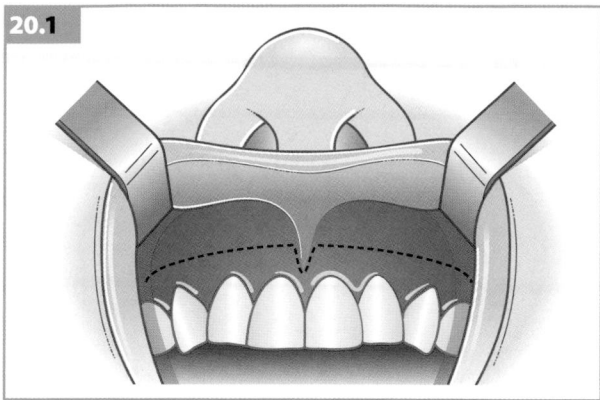

20.1 Sublabial incision.

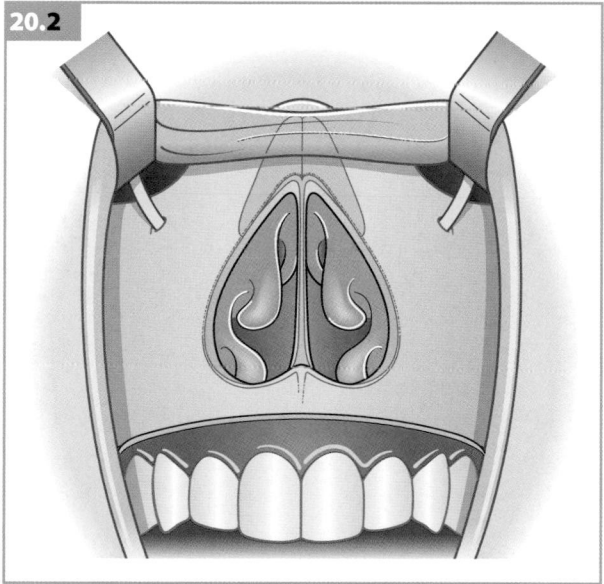

20.2 Exposure of the midface.

✪ Surgeon's tip

Leave a cuff of mucosa on the maxilla to facilitate easier suturing of the intraoral incision at the end of the procedure.

✪✪ Surgeon's tip

Take extra care to avoid damage to the infraorbital nerve as it exits the infraorbital foramen bilaterally.

✪✪✪ Surgeon's tip

16 mg of dexamethasone is used to reduce postoperative swelling.

21 Fine needle aspiration cytology

PROCEDURAL STEPS

1 **Equipment preparation**
2 **Fine needle aspirate**
3 **Slide preparation**

Equipment required:
- 20 ml syringe
- Green – 21 gauge needle
- Syringe mount
- Alcohol wipe
- Cotton wool
- Plaster
- 4 glass slides
- Slide carrier box
- Pencil
- Specimen pot with formalin

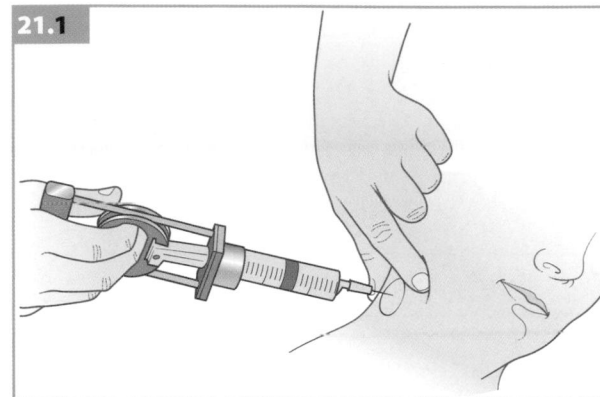

21.1 *Fine needle aspiration.*

PROCEDURE

1 Equipment preparation
Label glass slides with the patient's details using pencil. Label the specimen pot. Load syringe and needle into mount if using one.

2 Fine needle aspirate
Clean the skin with an alcohol wipe. Fix the mass between thumb and index finger. Insert the needle into the middle of the mass, and fully withdraw the plunger. Sample tissue by moving the needle tip around a few millimetres within the mass (**21.1**). Withdraw the needle, keeping the syringe plunger fully withdrawn. There is no need to repeat the procedure unless the first sample is contaminated with significant amounts of blood. If a separate specimen is required for microbiology, repeat the sampling technique with a second syringe and needle. Ensure haemostasis.

3 Slide preparation
Expel the contents of the syringe onto a glass slide, making sure the bevel of the needle is facing down, and spread the resulting specimen between two slides. Repeat with a second slide. Allow the four slides to dry before placing in the slide box and sealing the lid. Draw preservative solution into syringe and wash the contents back into the specimen pot. If required, also send samples for microbiology.

22 Lymph node biopsy

SURGICAL STEPS

1 **Positioning the patient**
2 **Incision**
3 **Excisional and incisional lymph node biopsy**
4 **Haemostasis and closure**
5 **Sample preparation**

PROCEDURE

1 Positioning the patient

Lymph node biopsy or excision may be performed under general or local anaesthetic. Position the operating table head-up. Turn the patient's head away from the operative side. Mark the incision over the lymph node, making use of relaxed skin tension lines, taking care to avoid the course of superficial nerves. Inject 10 ml 1% lignocaine with 1/200,000 adrenaline. Prepare the skin with betadine and drape the patient with a head drape (**22.1**, **22.2**). ✪

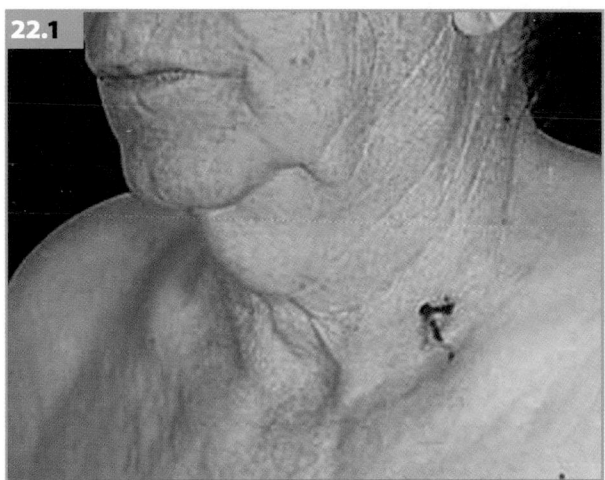

22.1 *Marking the biopsy site.*

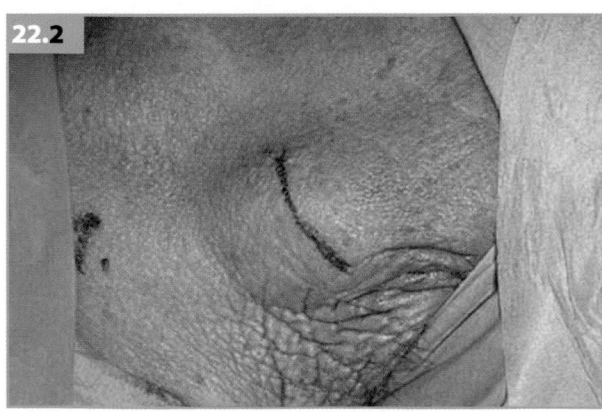

22.2 *Draping the biopsy site.*

✪ *Surgeon's tip* _____
*The lymph node to be biopsied should be marked preoperatively (**22.1**). If more than one lymph node is palpable, consider other factors which may make the biopsy easier, e.g. depth of lymph node, course of adjacent nerves, in particular the marginal mandibular branch of the facial nerve, accessory nerve, and great auricular nerve.*
_____

2 Incision

Incise skin, subcutaneous fat and platysma with a 10 blade. Palpate the node to localise it, and using McIndoe scissors and nontoothed forceps, gently dissect until you reach the surface of the lymph node. Retract the sternocleidomastoid muscle if necessary. A small self-retainer may be used (**22.3**).

3 Excisional and incisional lymph node biopsy

If possible, excise the whole lymph node (**22.4**). Using McIndoe scissors, dissect close to the surface of the lymph node to avoid damaging surrounding structures. Use diathermy to the vascular pedicle. If excision of the node is impossible, use cutting diathermy to remove a wedge of tissue. ✪

4 Haemostasis and closure

Ensure haemostasis. Occasionally a suction drain may be necessary. Close deep cervical fascia and platysma with 2/0 vicryl, and use 3/0 prolene or staples for skin (**22.5**).

5 Sample preparation

The specimen should be divided into dry and formalin samples as required; be guided by instructions and preferences from your local histopathology and haematology departments. Microbiology samples may also be provided at this time.

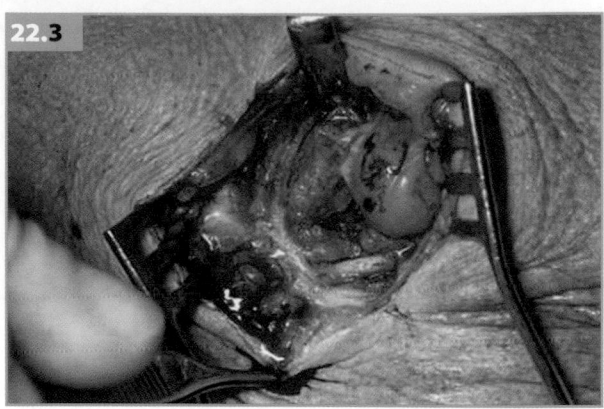

22.3 *Exposure of the lymph node.*

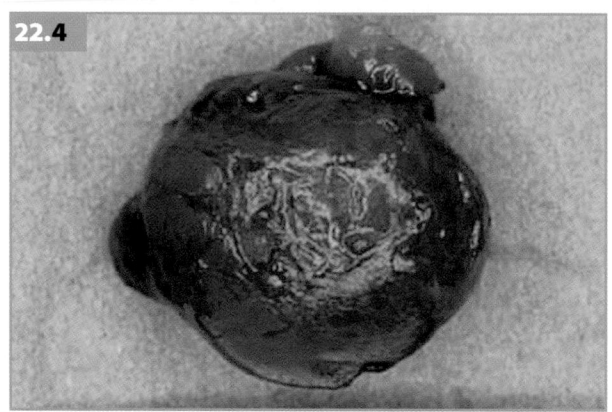

22.4 *Whole lymph node biopsy.*

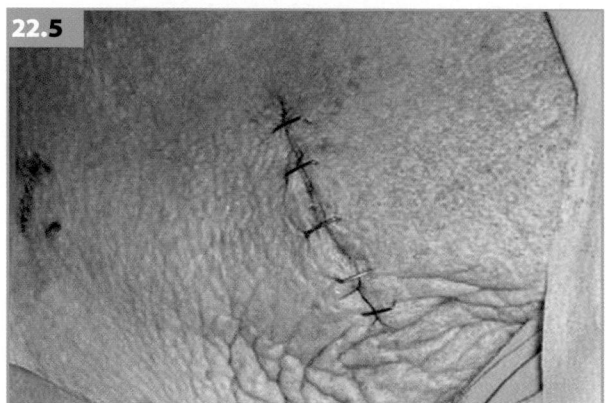

22.5 *Skin closure.*

✪ *Surgeon's tip* _____

To preserve the architecture of the lymph node, avoid handling the tissue directly. Use Allis forceps or nontoothed forceps on the lymph node capsule to prevent tissue damage.

23 Tonsillectomy and adenoidectomy

Tonsillectomy

SURGICAL STEPS

1 **Positioning the patient**
2 **Inserting a Boyle–Davis gag**
3 **Dissecting the tonsils**
4 **Haemostasis**

PROCEDURE

1 Positioning the patient
Position the patient's head close to the end of the operating table. Place a sandbag under the patient's shoulders to extend the neck. Drape the patient's head, leaving the nose and mouth exposed.

2 Inserting a Boyle–Davis gag
Ensure that the endotracheal tube is secured in the midline. Inspect the oral cavity for loose or damaged teeth. Select an appropriately-sized tongue depressor. Hold the Boyle–Davis gag with your right hand and open the patient's mouth using the index finger and thumb of the left hand. Insert the Boyle–Davis gag along the endotracheal tube and secure the tooth guard over the upper incisors. The endotracheal tube should rest in the groove of the tongue depressor and the tongue should lie in the midline. Gently open the Boyle–Davis gag taking care to avoid injury to the lips. Position the Boyle–Davis gag on Draffin rods to achieve a good view of the tonsils, and suction any secretions from the oral cavity (**23.1**). ✪

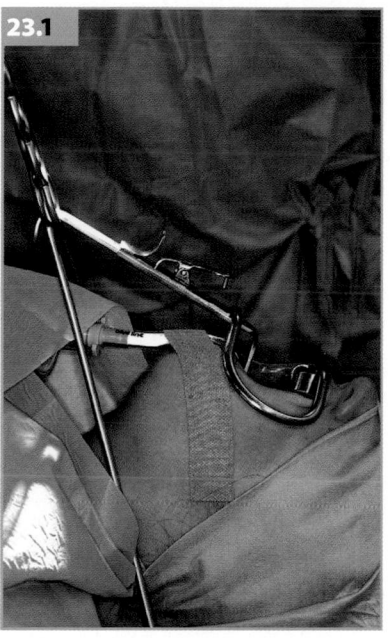

23.1 *Inserting a Boyle–Davis gag.*

✪ *Surgeon's tip* _____
If the patient is edentulous, use a gauze swab over the upper gum to protect it from damage and to anchor the gag.
_____

✪ *Surgeon's tip* _____
If operating on a patient with Down's syndrome, take care with neck positioning as there is a higher incidence of atlanto–axial instability.
_____

✪ Surgeon's tip

Avoid dissecting the tongue base which can lead to troublesome bleeding.

✪✪ Surgeon's tip

Occasionally bleeding may be severe. Apply an haemostatic agent (e.g. Surgicel®) in the tonsillar fossae and suture posterior and anterior tonsillar pillars together with interrupted 2/0 vicryl.

✪✪ Surgeons's tip

Once the surgeon is familiar with cold steel dissection, bipolar diathermy can be used as an alternative technique. Other techniques include coblation and laser dissection, and in the USA monopolar diathermy is sometimes used.

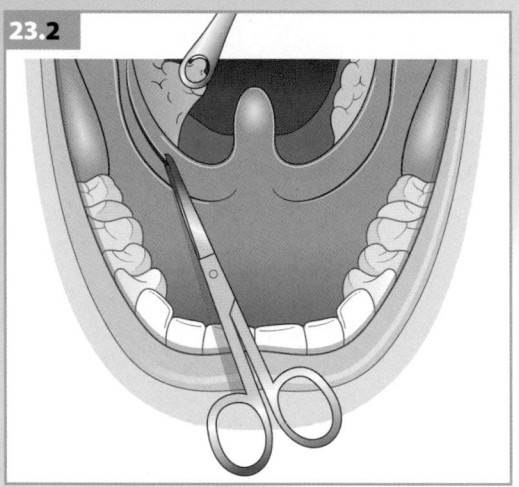

23.2

23.2 *Curved incision.*

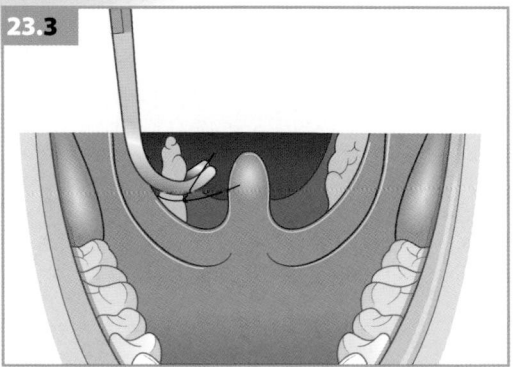

23.3

23.3 *Haemostasis.*

3 Dissecting the tonsils

Using tonsillar forceps (Dennis Brown) retract the tonsil medially. Use scissors to make a curved mucosal incision approximately 2 mm lateral to the edge of the anterior tonsillar pillar at the level of the upper tonsillar pole (**23.2**). Extend the incision inferiorly towards the tongue base and medially towards the uvula, taking care not to tear it. Using scissor dissection, identify the superior tonsillar pole, and retract the superior pole medially and inferiorly with tonsillar forceps. Use a Gwynne Evans dissector to dissect in a plane between the tonsillar capsule and the pharyngeal wall, avoiding trauma to the muscles of the pharyngeal wall. Injury to pharyngeal muscles causes increased risk of bleeding and postoperative pain. ✪

4 Haemostasis

Use a curved Negus forceps to clamp the lower tonsillar pole and a 2/0 vicryl tie to ligate it. Ligate bleeding points using straight Negus forceps and ties (**23.3**). Pack the tonsillar fossae with a tonsillar swab while continuing with the contralateral side. This will usually control minor bleeding.

Remove tonsillar swabs and check for bleeding. Ensure haemostasis is achieved before removing the Boyle–Davis gag.

Suction any blood from the postnasal space using a fine suction catheter passed through the nose. Relax the Boyle–Davis gag for 3 minutes. Ensure there is no bleeding. Repeat haemostasis, if necessary. Remove the mouth gag, taking care not to displace the endotracheal tube. ✪✪

Adenoidectomy

SURGICAL STEPS

1 **Positioning the patient**
2 **Inserting a Boyle–Davis gag**
3 **Suction diathermy adenoidectomy**

PROCEDURE

1 Positioning the patient

Position the patient's head close to the end of the operating table. Place the patient flat on the table. Drape the patient's head leaving the nose and mouth exposed. ✪

2 Inserting a Boyle–Davis gag

As for tonsillectomy. ✪✪

3 Suction diathermy adenoidectomy

Retract the soft palate using fine suction catheters passed through the nose (**23.4**). Using a laryngeal mirror, inspect the postnasal space.

Use the suction diathermy wand to ablate the adenoidal tissue, under direct vision with the mirror (**23.5**). Avoid diathermy to the lateral wall as this causes injury to Eustachian tube orifices and potential scarring. Aim to see clearly the vomer at the end of the procedure. Use a wet tonsil swab to clear any debris and dissipate the heat, and after removal ensure the postnasal space is dry with the mirror. ✪✪✪

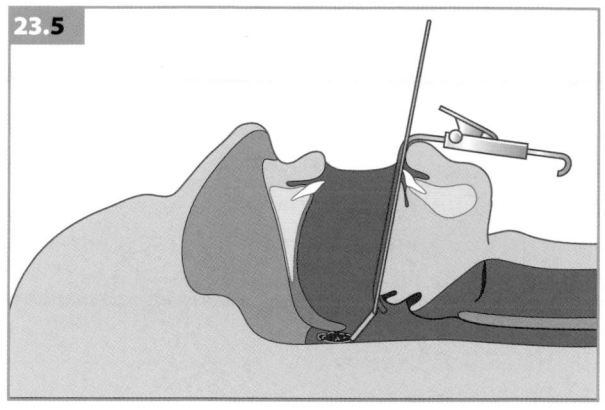

23.5 *Visualising adenoids using laryngeal mirror.*

✪ Surgeon's tip ――――――――
Avoid overextension of the neck, as this causes increased risk of damage to posterior pharyngeal wall structures.

✪✪ Surgeon's tip ――――――――
Ensure the uvula is not bifid, and palpate the palate to exclude anatomical abnormalities such as submucosal cleft palate.

✪✪✪ Surgeon's tip ――――――――
Antibiotics are advised following suction diathermy adenoidectomy, to avoid an infection in the sloughy healing bed and halitosis.

✪✪✪ Surgeon's tip ――――――――
A curette can be used as an alternative method for adenoidectomy

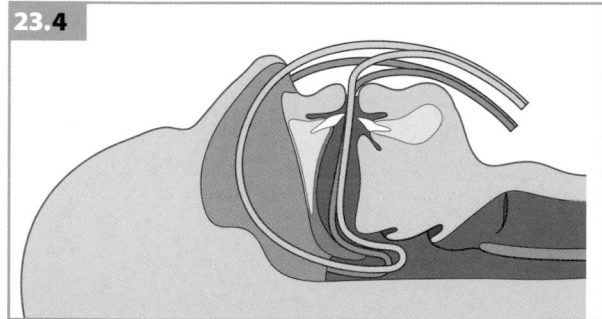

23.4 *Retraction of soft palate.*

24 Uvulopalatoplasty

SURGICAL STEPS

1 **Positioning the patient**
2 **Inserting a Boyle–Davis gag and local anaesthetic and adrenaline infiltration**
3 **Dissection**
4 **Haemostasis**

PROCEDURE

1 Positioning the patient

Position the patient's head close to the end of the operating table. Place a sandbag under the patient's shoulders to extend the neck. Drape the patient's head leaving the nose and mouth exposed.

2 Inserting a Boyle–Davis gag and local anaesthetic and adrenaline infiltration

Ensure that the endotracheal tube is secured in the midline. Inspect the oral cavity for loose or damaged teeth. Select an appropriately-sized tongue depressor. Hold the Boyle–Davis gag with your right hand and open the patient's mouth using the index finger and thumb of your left hand. Insert the Boyle–Davis gag along the endotracheal tube and secure the tooth guard over the upper incisors. The endotracheal tube should rest in the groove of the tongue depressor and the tongue should lie in the midline.

Gently open the Boyle–Davis gag taking care to avoid injury to the lips. Position the Boyle–Davis gag on Draffin rods (**24.1**) to achieve a good view of the palate and tonsils. Alternatively, a Mayo stand can be used. Suction any secretions from the oral cavity. Inject local anaesthetic and adrenaline (2 dental cartridges of 2% lignocaine and 1/80,000 adrenaline) to the palate.

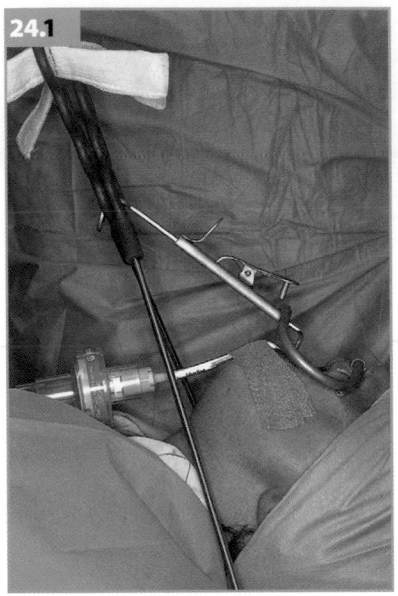

24.1 *Inserting a Boyle–Davis gag.*

3 Dissection

If the tonsils are present, they are removed (*see 23 – Tonsillectomy and adenoidectomy*). Palatal resection can be performed with cutting diathermy, CO_2, Nd-YAG, or KTP laser. If using laser, routine laser precautions must be taken and the face, oropharynx, and nasopharynx should be protected with wet swabs. (*See 29 – Microlaryngoscopy and laser use, for more details of laser safety.*)

Palpate the junction of the hard and soft palate. Using diathermy or laser, mark the superior limit of your dissection by measuring 25% of the length of the soft palate on either side of the uvula (**24.2**). Hold the palatal tissue under tension with Dennis Brown forceps. Excise a wedge of soft palate up to the marked point, including a strip of anterior tonsillar pillar. Trim half the length of the uvula (**24.3**, **24.4**). ✪

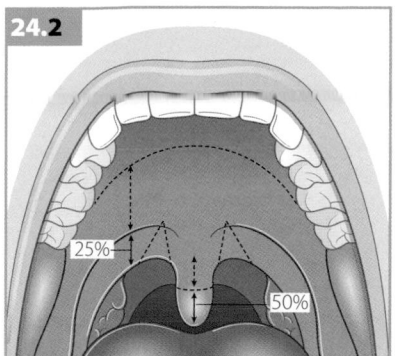

24.2 *Measuring limit of dissection from junction of the hard and soft palates.*

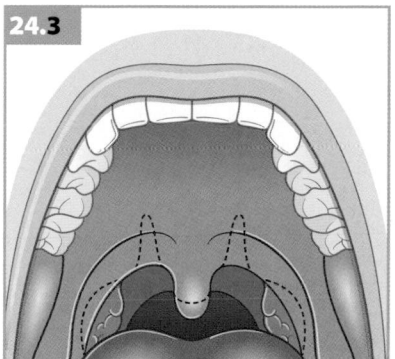

24.3 *Dissection lines marked.*

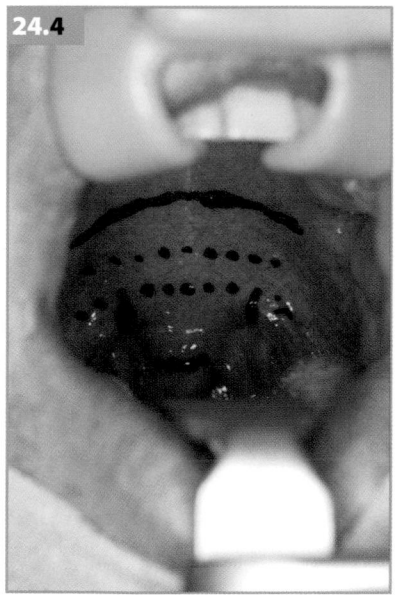

24.4 *Intraoperative view of dissection lines.*

4 Haemostasis

Ensure haemostasis and suture mucosal edges of uvula with 2/0 vicryl. Suction any blood from the postnasal space using a fine suction catheter passed through the nose. Remove the Boyle–Davis gag, taking care not to displace the endotracheal tube.

✪ *Surgeon's tip* _____

Many variations on the basic technique for dissection are described. The authors use a variation of the Kamani technique.

✪ *Surgeon's tip* _____

The uvula arteries may retract and cause troublesome bleeding during dissection of the palate. Avoid this by initially dissecting the palatal mucosa, and then use monopolar diathermy to cauterise tissue in the region of the uvula artery.

25 Tracheostomy

Adult elective tracheostomy

SURGICAL STEPS

1 **Positioning the patient**
2 **Marking and local anaesthetic**
3 **Incision**
4 **Separating the strap muscles**
5 **Dividing the thyroid isthmus**
6 **Checking the equipment**
7 **Tracheotomy and insertion of the tube**
8 **Securing the tube, closure, and dressing**

PROCEDURE

1 Positioning the patient

Position the patient's head close to the end of the operating table on a head ring. Place a sandbag under the patient's shoulders to extend the neck. Position the operating table head-up. Ensure an endotracheal tube is positioned superiorly and that the anaesthetist has access to it. Prepare the skin with aqueous betadine from chin superiorly to nipples inferiorly, and tie a head drape. ✪

2 Marking and local anaesthetic

Mark a 5 cm transverse skin crease incision midway between the sternal notch and cricoid ring. Inject 20 ml of local anaesthetic in the form of 0.5% lignocaine with 1/200,000 adrenaline (**25.1**). ✪✪

3 Incision

Using a 10 blade, incise skin, subcutaneous fat, and platysma, until you reach the anterior jugular veins. Divide and ligate the anterior jugular veins with 2/0 vicryl. Continue dissecting until you reach the level of strap muscles (**25.2**). Apply a self-retainer.

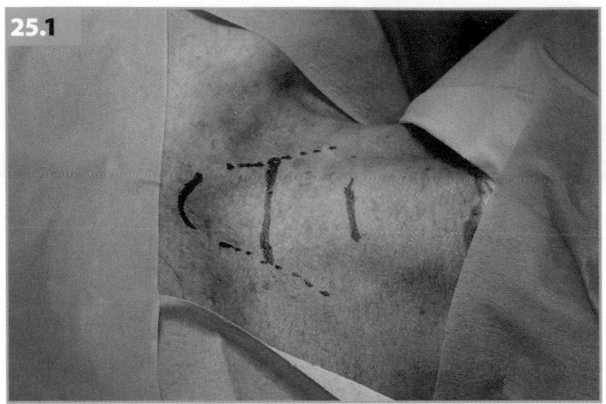

25.1 *Marking for tracheostomy.*

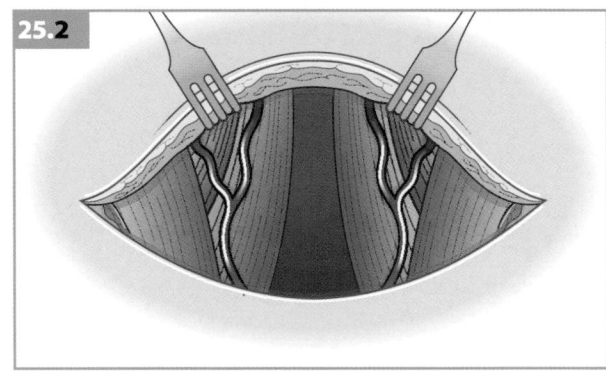

25.2 *Dividing the anterior jugular veins and exposing the strap muscles.*

✪ **Surgeon's tip**

Always assess a patient's neck preoperatively, and consider any factors which may affect ease of access to trachea:
- *Obesity.*
- *Limited neck extension.*
- *Short neck.*
- *Previous neck surgery or radiotherapy.*

✪ **Surgeon's tip**

In obese patients, use a tape passing round the chin up to the head of the table, to lift redundant skin and fat out of the operative field.

4 Separating the strap muscles

Separate the strap muscles in the midline using McIndoe scissors. Using a Lahey swab, expose the thyroid isthmus. Insert two Langenbeck retractors under the sternothyroid muscle (**25.3**).

5 Dividing the thyroid isthmus

Using a heavy clip, separate the isthmus of thyroid from the underlying trachea. Insert clips and divide the isthmus as shown (**25.4–25.6**). Transfix the isthmus with 2/0 vicryl. ✪✪✪

✪✪ **Surgeon's tip**

Tracheostomy may occasionally need to be performed under local anaesthetic (LA) in an urgent clinical setting. Initially instil LA and adrenaline into the skin and subcutaneous tissues, and infiltrate into the deeper tissues as you progress. Before tracheal fenestration inject LA into the trachea.

✪✪✪ **Surgeon's tip**

It is the authors' practice to divide the thyroid isthmus using monopolar cutting diathermy.

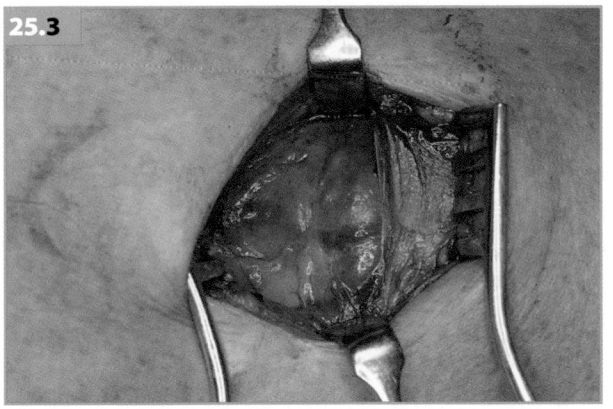

25.3 *Separating the strap muscles.*

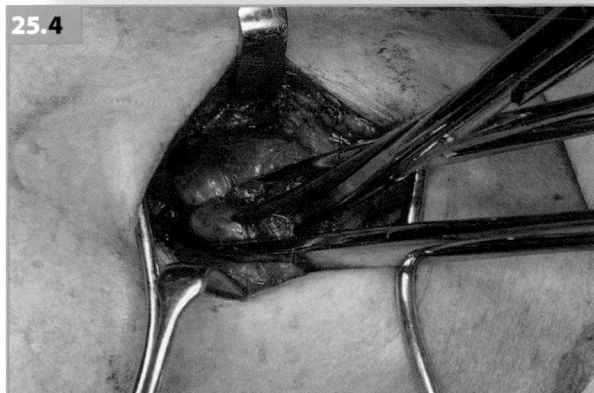

25.4–25.6 *Dividing the thyroid isthmus.*

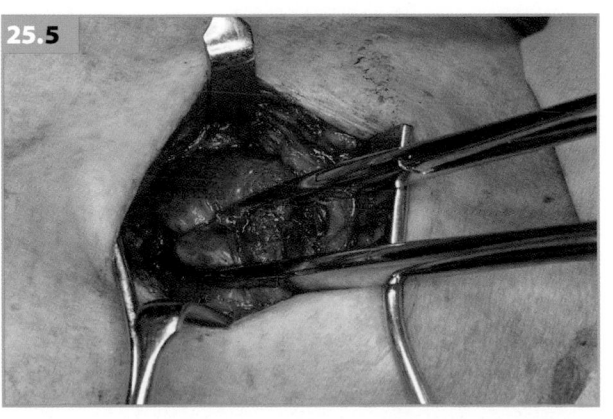

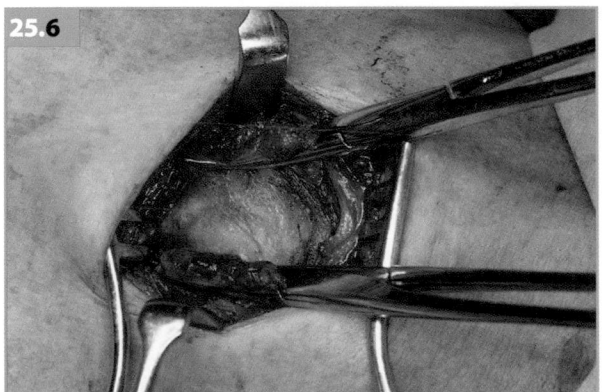

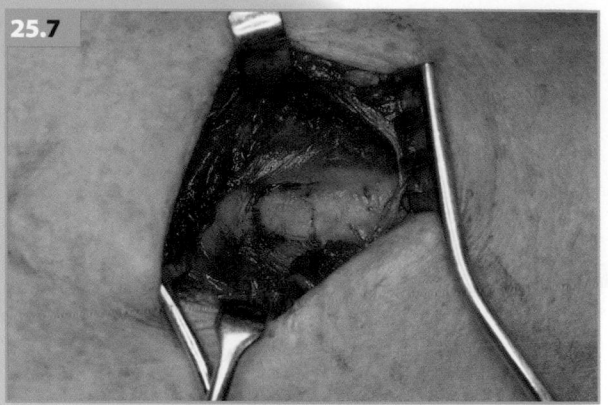

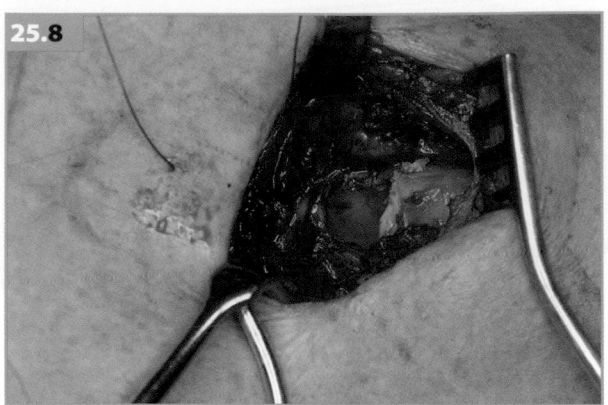

25.7, 25.8 *Tracheotomy.*

✪ **Surgeon's tip** ——————
*Use stay sutures between the tracheal window and skin to ensure unrestricted access in the event of the tracheostomy tube being dislodged (**25.9**).*

✪✪ **Surgeon's tip**——————
It is the authors' practice to suture the flange of the tracheostomy tube to the skin using 0 nylon for added security.

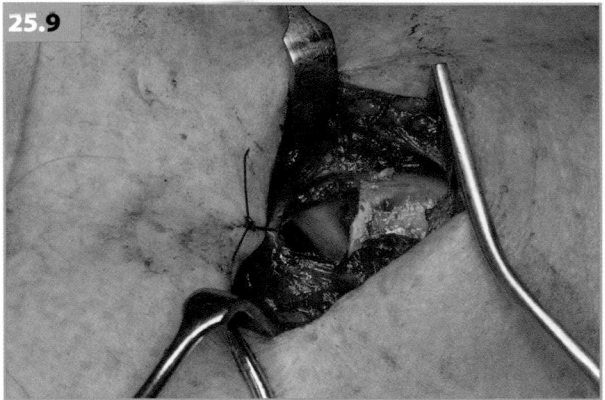

25.9 *Stay suture between trachea and skin.*

6 Checking the equipment

Check the tracheostomy tube size is correct and test the cuff with 20 ml air or saline; check suction is available. Insert the obturator and apply aqueous gel to the tip. If a double lumen tracheostomy is to be used, ensure that a nonfenestrated inner tube is available. Have spare tracheostomy tubes, tracheal dilators, and suction available.

7 Tracheotomy and insertion of the tube

Warn the anaesthetist that you are ready to perform the tracheotomy. Using a new 11 blade, make a fenestration in the trachea, between the second and third tracheal rings (**25.7**, **25.8**). Use heavy forceps to hold the tracheal tissue. Ask the anaesthetist to slowly withdraw the endotracheal

tube, until the tip is only just visible. Suction the secretions. Insert the tracheostomy tube and replace the obturator with the nonfenestrated inner tube. Inflate the cuff. Check the patient is adequately ventilated. ✪

8 Securing the tube, closure, and dressing

Remove retractors and self-retainers and check haemostasis. Loosely close skin with 2/0 prolene. Secure the tracheostomy tube with tapes and insert lyofoam dressing. Check tapes are tight – it should be possible to insert two fingers between the tapes and skin when the neck has been returned to neutral position. ✪✪

Paediatric elective tracheostomy

Details differing from adults:
- If you are unable to palpate the cricoid, feel for the hyoid bone.
- No local anaesthetic is required.
- De-fat the neck with a cutting diathermy needle.
- Separate strap muscles with a cutting diathermy needle.
- Divide the thyroid isthmus with bipolar diathermy.
- Insert two stay sutures from 2nd to 4th tracheal rings to control the tracheotomy slit: use prolene 4/0, clip the two loose suture ends and cut off the needle (**25.10**).
- Vertical incision in tracheal rings 2–4.

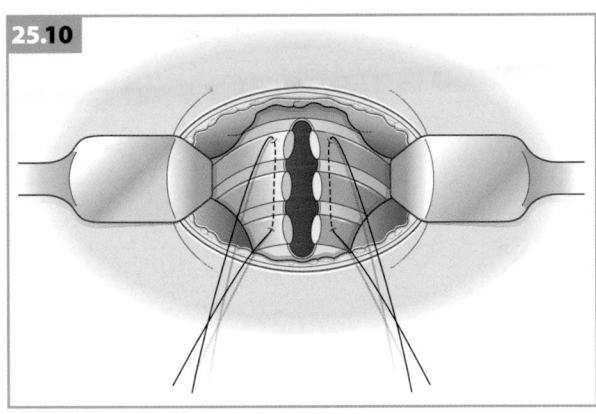

25.10 *Paediatric tracheotomy stay sutures.*

Emergency tracheostomy

Emergency tracheostomies are usually performed as a life-saving procedure. Make a longitudinal midline incision, using the fingers of the left hand to retract tissues, and palpate the trachea. Continue with an incision until the trachea is reached, and then make a vertical slit in the tracheal wall. Perform haemostasis after the airway has been secured.

26 Diagnostic procedures in the upper aerodigestive tract

Direct laryngoscopy (DL)

SURGICAL STEPS

1 Range of laryngoscopes
2 Assembling the equipment
3 Positioning the patient
4 Inserting the scope
5 Manipulation of the larynx
6 Biopsy or therapeutic procedure

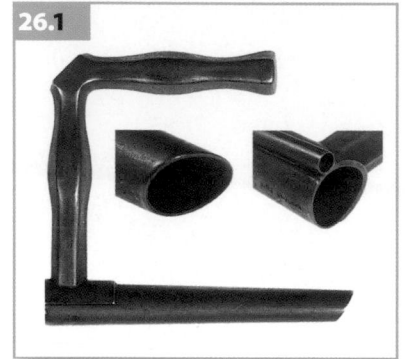

PROCEDURE

1 Range of laryngoscopes
Choose an appropriate laryngoscope from a range of scopes with different shapes, lengths, and luminal diameters to allow visualisation of all aspects of the larynx in all patients (**26.1–26.3**). ✪

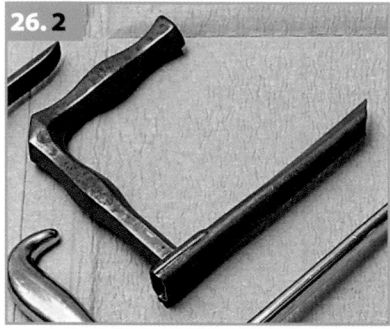

2 Assembling the equipment
You may need to use a single or a double light carrier, depending on the scope. Some laryngoscopes have a sliding blade which is used to allow large instruments or endotracheal tubes to be passed into the larynx. Assemble the laryngoscope and light carrier prior to laryngoscopy.

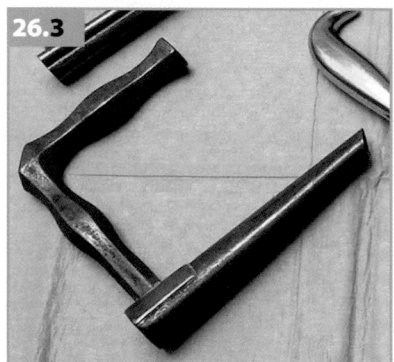

3 Positioning the patient
Position the patient supine on the operating table with a pillow under the shoulders, in the 'sniffing the morning air' position with the neck flexed towards the chest, and the head extended on the neck (**26.4**).

26.1–26.3 *Range of laryngoscopes.*

✪ **Surgeon's tip** _____
Discuss with the anaesthetist the choice of endotracheal tube (south facing RAE or microlaryngoscopy tube) and the side on which the tube should be secured.

✪ **Surgeon's tip** _____
The funnel-shaped designs, e.g. bouchayer, allow easier access for instruments and greater illumination with the microscope light.

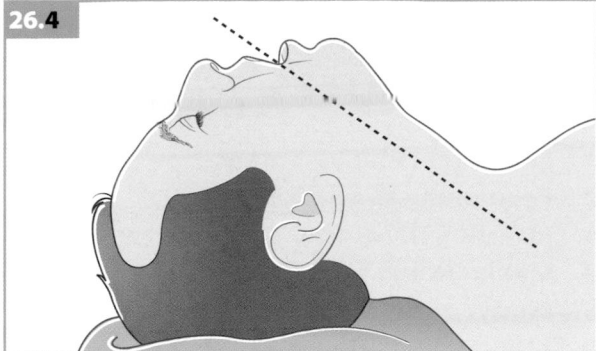

26.4 *Positioning the patient.*

✪✪ **Surgeon's tip** _____
Open the lower jaw by using the thumb to push it away from you, while simultaneously using the index and middle fingers to push the upper jaw. Avoid rotating the scope in the mouth or leaning on the dentition as a fulcrum. Use the thumb of the nondominant hand under the scope to prevent damage to the teeth.

✪✪✪ **Surgeon's tip** _____
A different scope may be needed to view the anterior commissure.

4 Inserting the scope

Protect the upper teeth with a mouth guard or a wet swab in edentulous patients. Lubricate the scope with a water-based gel.

Using your dominant hand, introduce the endoscope into the mouth, in the direction of the posterior pharyngeal wall. Using the other hand, keep the mouth open and protect the lips from damage (**26.5**, **26.6**). ✪✪

Advance the laryngoscope to the pharynx and uvula, being careful not to dislodge the endotracheal tube. Angle the scope to left and right and examine the tonsil fossae. Lift the scope as it is advanced in the midline pushing the tongue base up, with the endotracheal tube below the scope. Follow the endotracheal tube and advance the scope until you see the epiglottis. Examine the valleculae. Advance the scope under the epiglottis into the laryngeal inlet. Examine the supraglottic larynx, aryepiglottic folds, the infrahyoid laryngeal surface of the epiglottis, and the ventricular bands or false cords. Ensure you have a clear view of the whole of the larynx, vocal cords, and the anterior commissure. ✪✪✪

5 Manipulation of the larynx

Use external movement of the laryngeal framework to visualise all recesses of the larynx. Use 'cricoid pressure' to achieve a view of the anterior commissure.

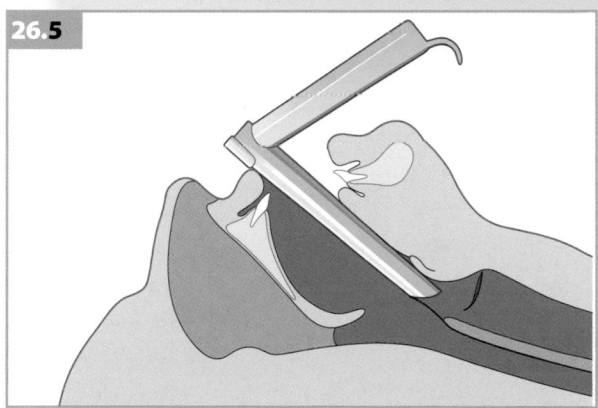

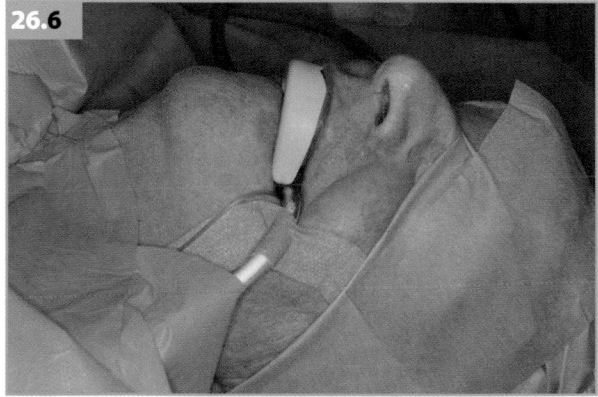

26.5, 26.6 *Insertion of the scope.*

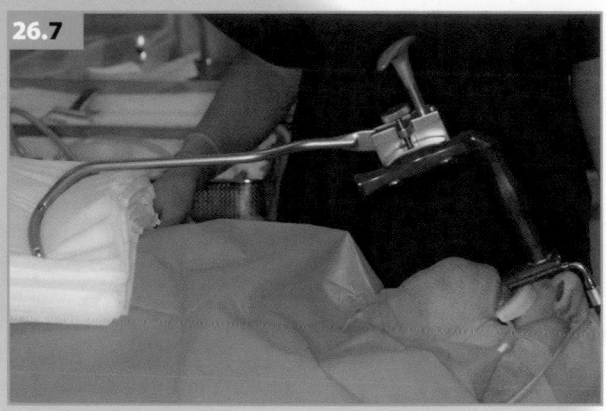

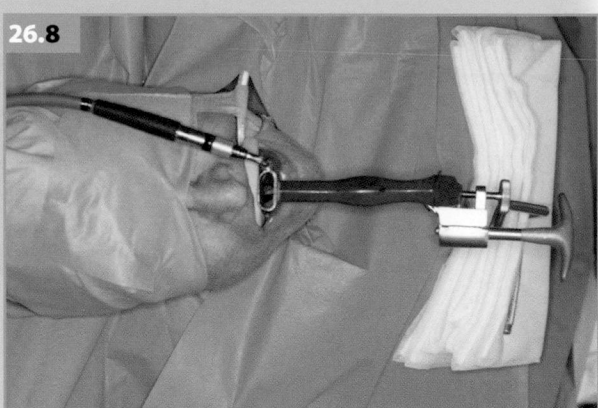

26.7, 26.8 *External stabiliser.*

6 Biopsy or therapeutic procedure

Hold the laryngoscope with your nondominant hand and take biopsies using the dominant hand. It is often useful to use an external stabiliser such as a suspension arm to free both hands for suction and biopsy forceps (**26.7, 26.8**). To view the laryngeal saccule, ventricle, and subglottic under surface of the vocal fold, use 0° and 90° Hopkins endoscope rods.

At the end of the procedure, withdraw the laryngoscope, taking care not to dislodge the endotracheal tube.

Direct pharyngoscopy (DP)

SURGICAL STEPS

1 **Equipment and assembly**
2 **Positioning the patient**
3 **Inserting the scope**
4 **Manipulation of the pharynx**
5 **Biopsy or therapeutic procedure**

PROCEDURE

1 Equipment and assembly

The pharyngoscope has a longer barrel than the laryngoscope and the upper or superior blade is longer (**26.9**). Assemble the pharyngoscope and double light carrier prior to pharyngoscopy.

2 Positioning the patient

Position as for a direct laryngoscopy. Further extension may be necessary to straighten the cervical oesophagus.

3 Inserting the scope

Protect the upper teeth with a mouth guard or a wet swab in edentulous patients. Lubricate the scope with a water-based gel. Insert the scope as in laryngoscopy. Follow the posterior pharyngeal wall further down the oropharynx toward the posterior hypopharyngeal wall, until you can see the postcricoid mucosa. The endotracheal tube should be above the scope at this point. ✪

4 Manipulation of the pharynx

Sweep the tip of the scope to one side and inspect the piriform fossa. Repeat on the other side. Now use the scope tip to lift the larynx forward and inspect the postcricoid mucosa as far down as cricopharyngeus muscle.

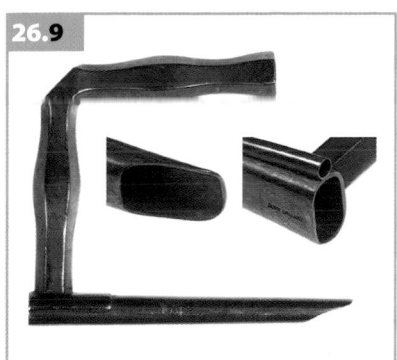

26.9 *Pharyngoscope.*

5 Biopsy or therapeutic procedure

Hold the pharyngoscope with your nondominant hand and take biopsies using the dominant hand, with long biopsy forceps or larger punch forceps. At the end of the procedure, withdraw the pharyngoscope, taking care not to dislodge the endotracheal tube. Palpate the tongue base and tonsil areas for any submucosal masses, and also palpate the neck for lymph nodes to complete the clinical staging.

Direct oesophagoscopy (DO)

SURGICAL STEPS

1 Range of oesophagoscopes
2 Equipment and assembly
3 Positioning the patient
4 Inserting the scope
5 Biopsy or therapeutic procedure

PROCEDURE

1 Range of oesophagoscopes

Oesophagoscopes are all similar shaped but have differing lengths and diameters. All oesophagoscopes have graduated markings indicating the distance of the tip of the oesophagoscope from the upper incisors (**26.10, 26.11**).

2 Equipment and assembly

Assemble the scope and light carrier. The light carrier may be single or double pronged or attached to a prism at the proximal end of the scope.

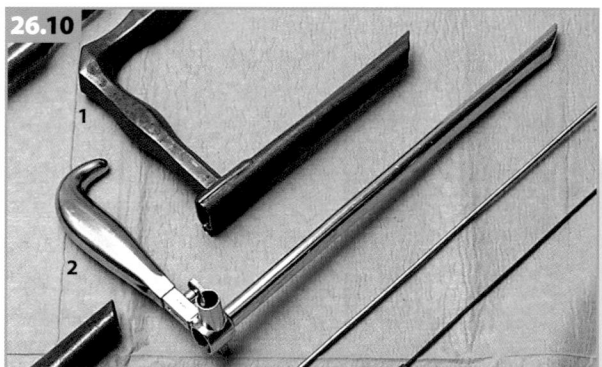

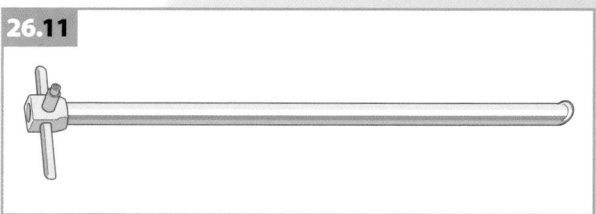

26.10, 26.11 *Oesophagoscopes. 1: laryngoscope; 2: oesophagoscope.*

✪ *Surgeon's tip* _____

Following the posterior pharyngeal wall can risk dislocating the arytenoids; an alternative technique is to follow the piriform fossa on one side towards the midline.

29 Microlaryngoscopy and laser use

Microlaryngoscopy

SURGICAL STEPS

1   **Range of laryngoscopes**
2   **Equipment assembly**
3   **Positioning the patient**
4   **Inserting the scope and jet ventilation**
5   **Manipulation of the larynx**
6   **Biopsy or therapeutic procedure,
    including laser**

PROCEDURE

1 Range of laryngoscopes
Choose an appropriate laryngoscope (*see 26 – Diagnostic procedures in the upper aerodigestive tract: Direct laryngoscopy*).

2 Equipment assembly
Ensure that if you will be using jet ventilation, the equipment is ready and has been checked by the anaesthetist. If you do not have access to jet ventilation, ask the anaesthetist to intubate with a size 5 microlaryngoscopy tube. If you are planning to use the laser, ensure that the anaesthetist inserts a laser resistant microlaryngoscopy tube. Make sure the microscope focal length is set to 400 mm.

3 Positioning the patient
Position the patient supine on the operating table with a pillow under the shoulders, in the 'sniffing the morning air' position (*see* **26.4**) with the neck flexed towards the chest, and the head extended on the neck.

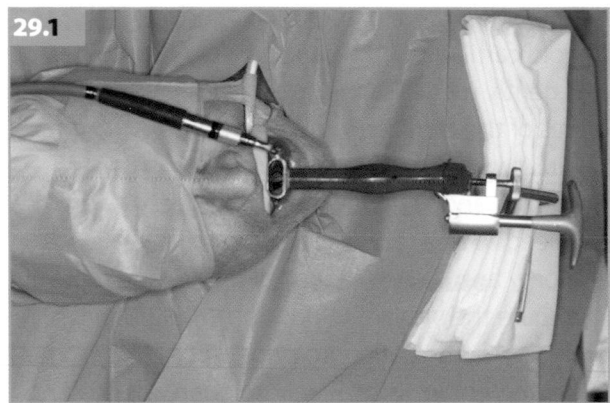

29.1 *Insertion of the laryngoscope.*

4 Inserting the scope and jet ventilation
Protect the upper teeth with a mouth guard or a wet swab in edentulous patients. Lubricate the scope with a water-based gel. Using your dominant hand, introduce the endoscope into the mouth, in the direction of the posterior pharyngeal wall, as for direct laryngoscopy. When you have a full view of the vocal folds, ask your assistant to attach the suspension apparatus, and secure the scope in the right position before bringing in the microscope (**29.1**); *see also* **28.1**.

Confirm with the anaesthetist that the patient is ventilating satisfactorily. At the end of the procedure, before the scope is withdrawn from the larynx, turn off the jet ventilator, and allow the anaesthetist to re-establish ventilation. (*See 27 – Paediatric microlaryngoscopy and bronchoscopy (MLB) foreign body removal*, and *28 – Phonosurgery, for pitfalls with jet ventilation.*) ✪

5 Manipulation of the larynx
Use external movement of the laryngeal framework to visualise all recesses of the larynx. Use 'cricoid pressure' to achieve a view of the anterior commissure.

6 Biopsy or therapeutic procedure, including laser

To view the laryngeal saccule, ventricle, and subglottic undersurface of the vocal fold, use 0° and 90° Hopkins endoscope rods.

The assistant should guide the instrument tips into the laryngoscope lumen while you continue looking down the microscope. Grip the instruments lightly, and use small movements of your fingers rather than the whole hand to achieve precise movement of the instruments. Using grasping forceps in one hand and curved scissors in the other, remove the lesion. Use an adrenaline-soaked neuropattie to achieve haemostasis.

At the end of the procedure, remove the suspension apparatus and withdraw the laryngoscope, taking care not to dislodge the endotracheal tube if in situ. ✪✪

Laser use in endoscopic procedures

Laser safety

The operating surgeon is responsible for laser safety. Before starting, you should check that:
- The doors to theatre are locked.
- All staff are wearing laser goggles.
- If appropriate, a laser-safe endotracheal tube is used.
- Wet swabs are placed over the patient's exposed skin.
- A jug of water is available to extinguish a laser fire.

Laser equipment

CO_2 laser may either be attached to the microscope and controlled via a laser micromanipulator (**29.2**), or delivered via a hand piece.

KTP laser is more commonly used in the nose and ear. It is delivered via a fibreoptic cable; take care not to damage the cable when setting up the hand piece. The end of the cable should be cut at right angles using the cable cutter, to produce a sharp point for safe and accurate delivery.

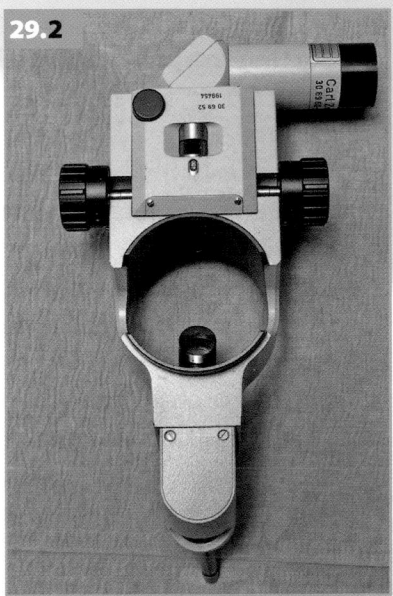

29.2 *Microscope/laser micromanipulator.*

✪ **Surgeon's tip** _____

Always remember that the facial nerve will be found at the same depth as the insertion of the posterior belly of digastric muscle.

✪ **Surgeon's tip** _____

If unable to identify the facial nerve, alternative techniques include identifying the distal branches and tracing in a retrograde fashion back to the main nerve trunk, or performing a mastoidectomy and tracing the nerve upwards.

✪✪ **Surgeon's tip** _____

The authors advocate the technique of partial superficial parotidectomy for benign disease. In this technique, the tumour is removed with a 1 cm cuff of normal parotid tissue, rather than removing the whole superficial lobe, as traditionally described.

✪✪ **Surgeon's tip** _____

Always use the mosquito clip in a direction parallel to the direction of the facial nerve to avoid injury to the nerve.

4 Facial nerve identification

Using 15 blade or iris pointed scissors, dissect the anterior margin of the sternomastoid muscle superiorly, as far as the mastoid process. Expose the perichondrium of tragus and the anterior wall of the external auditory canal and connect the incisions. Dissect medially to the anterior border of the sternomastoid muscle until the posterior belly of the digastric muscle is identified.

Dissect the loose connective tissue between the parotid gland and mastoid bone using a mosquito clip until you identify the tympano-mastoid suture. A small amount of fat separates the facial nerve from the mastoid bone. Using a mosquito clip, expose the facial nerve (**32.4**, **32.5**). ✪

5 Superficial parotidectomy

Using a mosquito clip, follow the main trunk of the facial nerve and its two main divisions. Insert the mosquito clip parallel to the direction of the nerve. Lift the parotid gland away from the nerve and cut between the tips of the mosquito clip with a 15 blade. Repeat this technique as you follow the main trunk of the facial nerve and its branches. Remove the superficial part of the parotid gland which contains the tumour (**32.6**, **32.7**).

Use bipolar diathermy for haemostasis, but avoid manipulating the facial nerve. ✪✪

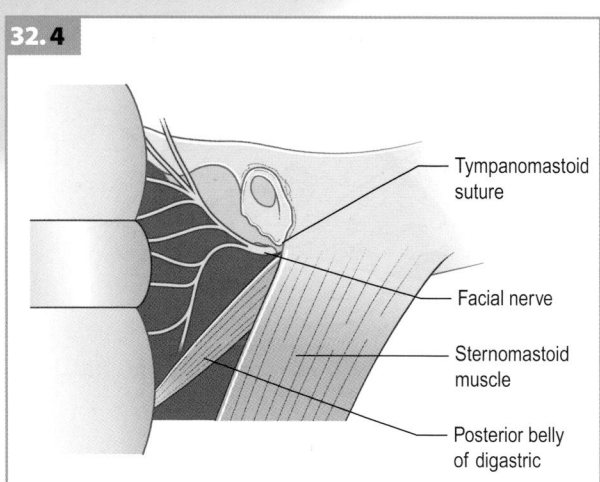

32.4 *Anatomy of the facial nerve.*

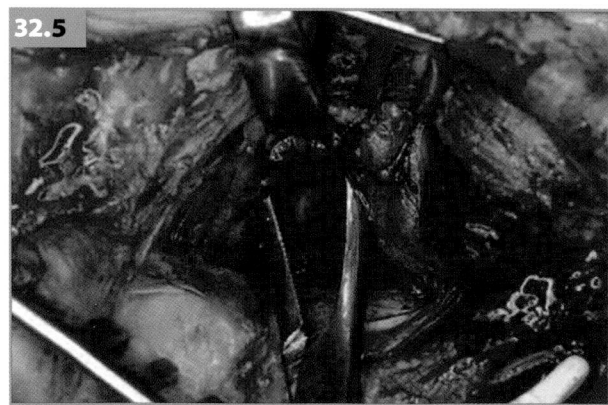

32.5 *Exposure of the facial nerve.*

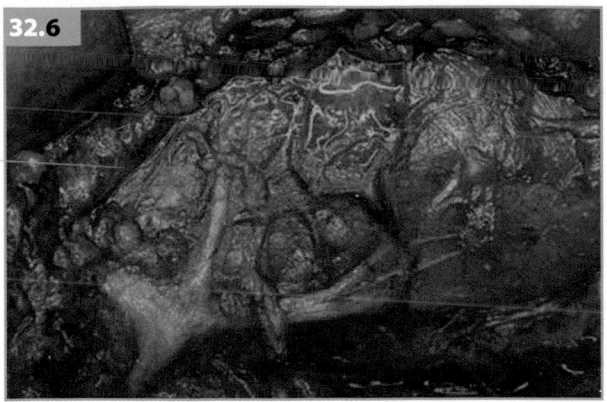

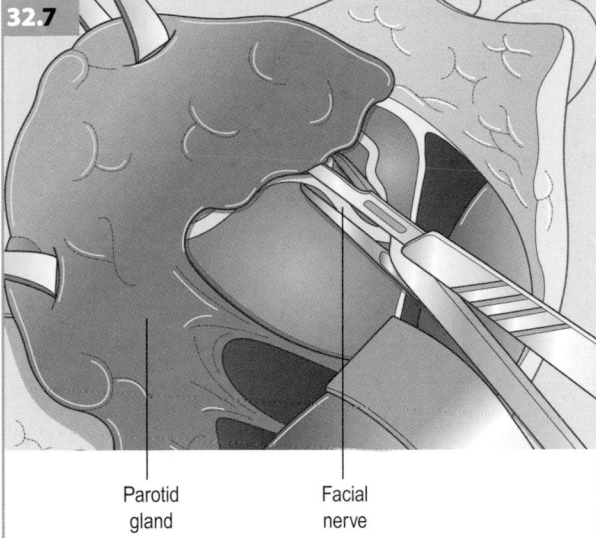

Parotid gland   Facial nerve

32.6, 32.7 *Removing the superficial part of the parotid gland.*

6 Sternomastoid flap reconstruction

Fill the parotid gland defect using a superiorly-based sternomastoid pedicle muscle flap. Use iris scissors to expose the superficial aspect of sternomastoid muscle. Then create a flap using bipolar cutting diathermy. Stitch the distal end of the pedicled flap into the parotid defect using 3/0 vicryl. ✪✪✪

7 Closure and dressing

A small vacuum drain is inserted superficial to the sternomastoid flap. Close the preauricular skin incision with 5/0 prolene (**32.8**). Use skin clips to close postauricular and hairline incisions. Place a piece of cotton wool in the external auditory meatus, a paraffin-impregnated dressing such as Jelonet® dressing over the incision, and apply a head bandage. ✪✪✪✪

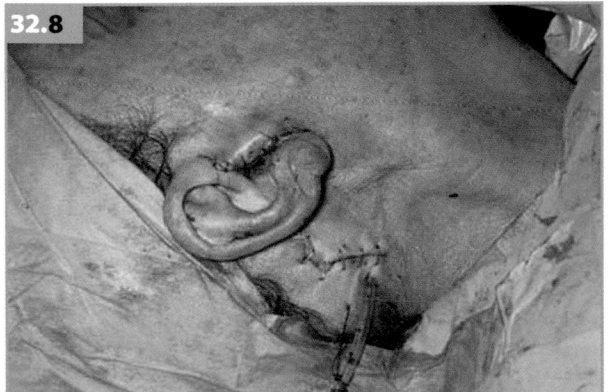

32.8 *Closure of the preauricular skin incision with vacuum drain in place.*

✪✪✪ ***Surgeon's tip***———
Using a sternomastoid flap to fill the parotid defect improves the cosmetic outcome and reduces the incidence of Frey's syndrome.

✪✪✪✪ ***Surgeon's tip***———
The author advocates the use of 16 mg intravenous dexamethasone just before the end of the procedure to limit post-operative oedema.

33 Thyroglossal cyst excision (Sistrunk's procedure)

SURGICAL STEPS

1 **Positioning the patient**
2 **Incision**
3 **Mobilising the cyst and central neck dissection**
4 **Excision of the body of the hyoid bone**
5 **Haemostasis, drain, and closure**

PROCEDURE

1 Positioning the patient

Position the patient on the operating table head-up, with a sandbag under the shoulders and a head ring. Mark the incision with a sterile marker pen and inject 2% lignocaine with 1/80,000 adrenaline using a dental syringe.

2 Incision

Using a 10 blade, make a transverse skin crease incision at the upper margin of the cyst. Incise the skin and subcutaneous fat. Divide and ligate the anterior jugular veins if necessary.

3 Mobilising the cyst and central neck dissection

Using McIndoe scissors and nontoothed forceps, dissect the cyst from surrounding tissues, taking care not to rupture the capsule of the cyst. Superiorly follow the thyroglossal duct up to the level of the body of the hyoid. ✪

4 Excision of the body of the hyoid bone

Mobilise the body of the hyoid bone from its muscle attachments using cutting diathermy. Take care not to damage the thyrohyoid membrane which lies underneath the body of the hyoid bone. Grasp the central portion of the hyoid bone using Allis forceps. Separate the middle third of the hyoid bone using bone cutters (**33.1**).

Place your index finger in the oral cavity and palpate the tongue base, pushing the tissues of the tongue base forwards (**33.2**). Using cutting diathermy, continue dissection superiorly, up to the level of the foramen caecum, removing a core of tongue musculature. Take care not to breach the oral mucosa. ✪✪

5 Haemostasis, drain, and closure

Following haemostasis, insert a size 10 FG vacuum drain. Close the skin in two layers using 3/0 vicryl and 4/0 prolene.

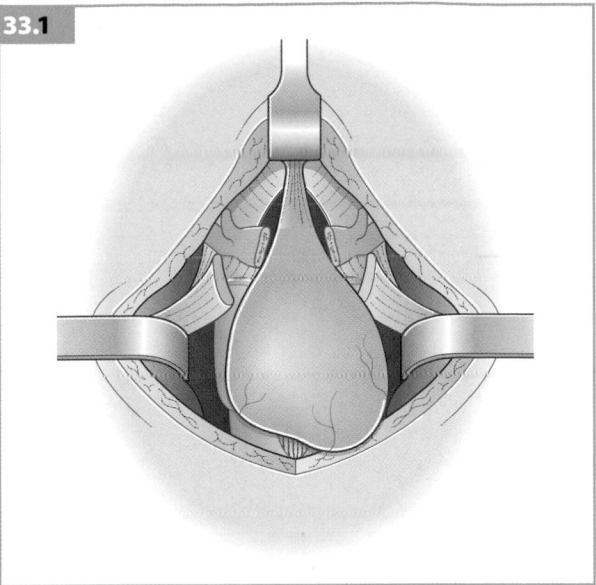

33.1 Excision of the body of the hyoid bone.

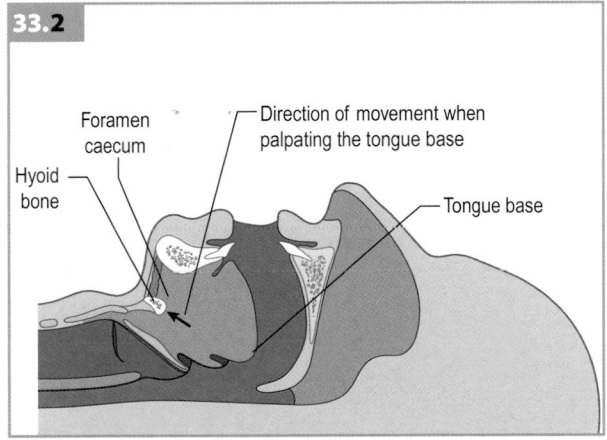

33.2 Excision of the core of suprahyoid musculature.

✪ *Surgeon's tip* _____

The senior author advocates resection of the whole anterior compartment of the neck from the level of the cyst to the body of the hyoid bone. This prevents the possibility of leaving any branches of the duct behind which may then lead to a recurrence.

✪✪ *Surgeon's tip* _____

Occasionally, the thyroglossal duct can extend onto the mucosal surface of the tongue base, or your dissection may breach the oral mucosa. If this occurs, is important to repair the defect to avoid development of an orocutaneous fistula.

34 Thyroidectomy

SURGICAL STEPS

1 **Positioning the patient and incision**
2 **Elevation of flaps**
3 **Mobilising the upper pole and localising the carotid gutter**
4 **Mobilising the lower pole and identifying the inferior parathyroid gland**
5 **Identifying the recurrent laryngeal nerve (RLN)**
6 **Division of Berry's ligament**
7 **Haemostasis and closure**

PROCEDURE

1 Positioning the patient and incision

Mark the skin crease incision with the patient sitting up in the anaesthetic room. Ensure the anaesthetist uses a RLN monitor endotracheal tube, and that correct positioning of the tube is confirmed. Position the patient on the operating table head-up, with a sandbag under the shoulders and a head ring. Infiltrate the skin with local anaesthetic in the form of 1% lignocaine with 1/200,000 adrenaline. Drape the patient with a head drape and side and body towels.

2 Elevation of flaps

Using a 10 blade incise the skin and platysma. Divide and ligate the anterior jugular veins if necessary. Elevate the subplatysmal flaps, superiorly to the level of thyroid cartilage and inferiorly to the suprasternal notch. Insert a Jolls retractor. Using McIndoe scissors and forceps, divide the deep investing layer of cervical fascia and strap muscles in the midline. The strap muscles should be preserved, unless access is restricted. ✪

3 Mobilising the upper pole and localising the carotid gutter

Identify the carotid gutter and ligate the middle thyroid vein.

The gutter is carefully dissected to avoid a nonrecurrent laryngeal nerve, seen in 1% of cases, on the right side. Mobilise the upper pole, by applying traction on the strap muscles and the carotid sheath using Langenbeck retractors. Place an Allis retractor on the superior pole and retract it downwards and laterally to identify the external branch of superior laryngeal nerve (EBSLN) (**34.1, 34.2**). Inspect the posterior surface of the thyroid and identify the superior parathyroid gland (SPT), usually at the level of the cricothyroid junction (**34.3**). ✪✪

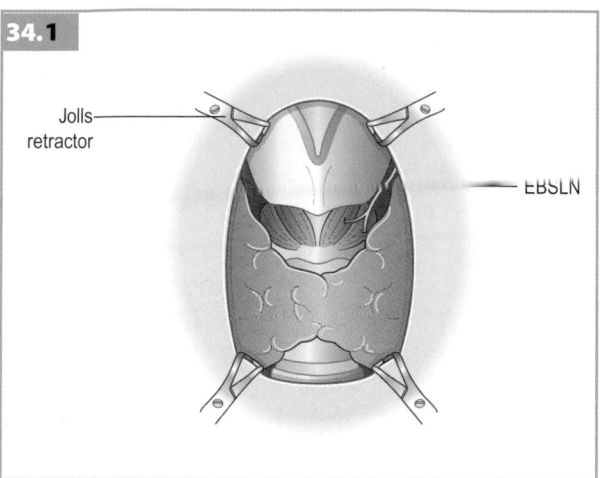

34.1 *Dissection of the superior pole. (EBSLN: external branch of superior laryngeal nerve)*

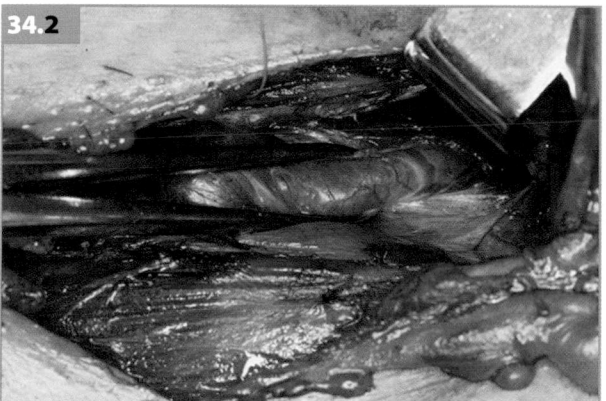

34.2 *Dissection of left superior pole.*

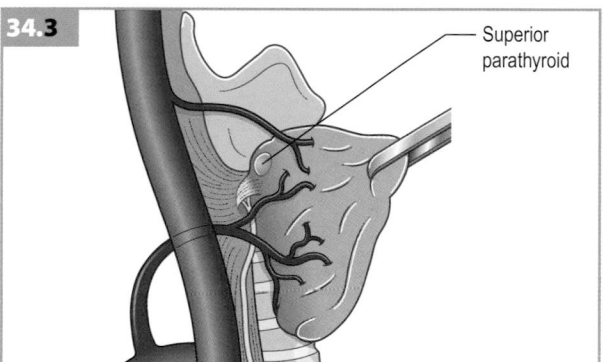

34.3 *Identification of the superior parathyroid gland.*

✪ **Surgeon's tip** ————

Division of the sternothyroid muscle superiorly close to its insertion to the thyroid cartilage is often a useful manoeuvre to allow greater exposure of the superior pole and identification of the external laryngeal nerve.

✪✪ **Surgeon's tip** ————

To avoid damage to the EBSLN be familiar with its course. Identify it within Joll's triangle and confirm its position with a nerve stimulator.

Aim to identify all the parathyroid glands. Perform extracapsular dissection to preserve the blood supply.

✪✪✪ **Surgeon's tip** ____
The right RLN is often more superficial than the left. The nerve may be displaced postero-laterally by Zuckerkandl's tubercle, a postero-lateral protrusion of thyroid tissue. On the right side, the nerve approaches the gland more obliquely.

✪✪✪ **Surgeon's tip** ____
The RLN is best identified low down. Here it forms one side of Beahr's triangle. Beahr's triangle is bounded by the RLN, inferior thyroid artery (ITA), and common carotid artery (34.4).

4 Mobilising the lower pole and identifying the inferior parathyroid gland

Identify the trachea below the isthmus in the midline and continue dissection through fascia to free the lower pole. Identify and ligate the inferior thyroid vein close to the gland. Inspect the posterior surface of the thyroid and identify the inferior parathyroid gland. When identified, gently peel back and preserve the gland. ✪✪

5 Identifying the RLN

Identify the nerve in the tracheo-oesophageal groove by careful dissection with a mosquito clip. Trace the nerve from below the gland to its entry into the larynx on both sides. Full dissection of the nerve is not required. It should not be 'skeletonised'. ✪✪✪ (34.4–34.7)

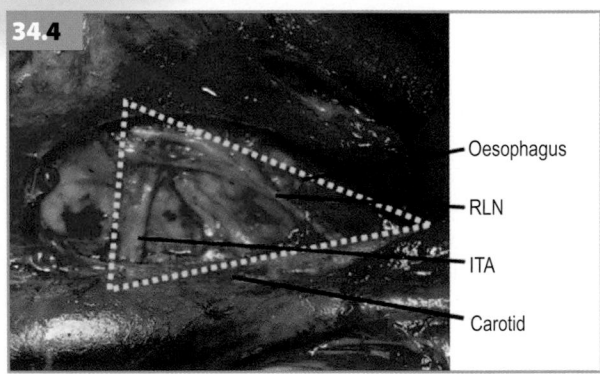

34.4

Oesophagus

RLN

ITA

Carotid

34.4 *Beahr's triangle showing position of recurrent laryngeal nerve.*

6 Division of Berry's ligament

Once you have identified the RLN, divide Berry's ligament. The lobe and isthmus are removed. In a hemithyroidectomy, the contralateral lobe is transfixed using 2/0 vicryl. For a total thyroidectomy, repeat the procedure on the contralateral side. Place an adrenaline (1/1,000) soaked tonsil swab in the wound, while you dissect the other side.

7 Haemostasis and closure

Ensure adequate haemostasis is achieved with a Valsalva manoeuvre and check the RLN and EBSLN. Place an absorbable haemostatic agent such as Surgicel® or Tisseel® in the thyroid bed. It is not the author's routine practice to insert drains. Close the strap muscles and platysma using 3/0 biosyn. Close skin with a 3/0 vicryl rapide suture and liquid skin adhesive such as Dermabond®. No dressing is applied to the incision.

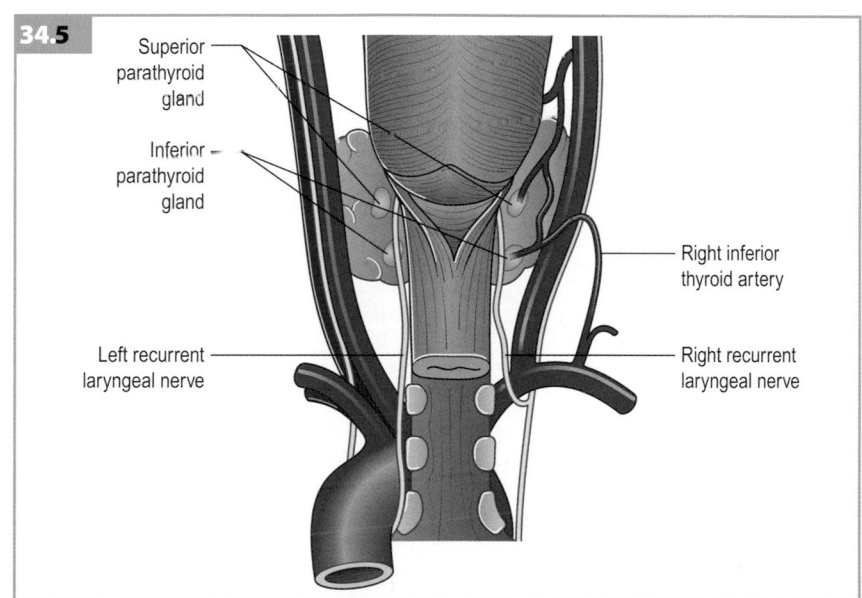

34.5 *Right and left recurrent laryngeal nerves, posterior view.*

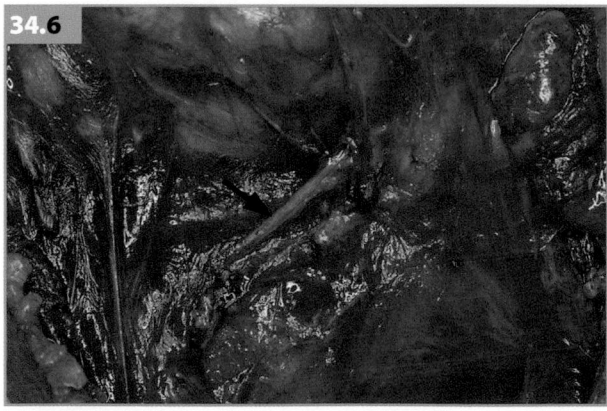

34.6 *Left recurrent laryngeal nerve (arrow).*

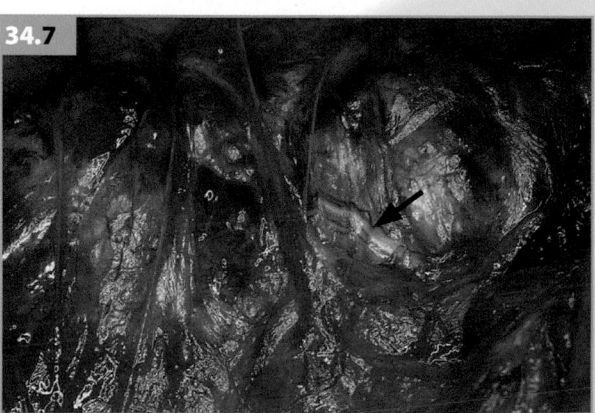

34.7 *Right recurrent laryngeal nerve (arrow).*

Neck dissection is divided into different types depending on which lymph nodes are dissected. *Table 35.1* shows the terminology used for these procedures. The technique used for a modified radical neck dissection type III (levels I–V) is described.

Modified radical neck dissection type III

SURGICAL STEPS

1 **Positioning the patient**
2 **Incision and subplatysmal flaps**
3 **Level I**
4 **Identifying XI**
5 **Level V**
6 **Levels II, III, IV**
7 **Haemostasis, drains, and closure**
8 **Orientating the specimen**

PROCEDURE

1 Positioning the patient
Position the patient with a sandbag under the shoulders and a head ring, and the operating table head-up. Use a marker pen to indicate the line of incision, which should run from the mastoid tip to the thyroid cartilage – the most commonly used incision is shown (**35.1**). An inferior limb will be required if level V is to be dissected. Ensure that the trifurcation of the incision does not overlie the carotid sheath. Infiltrate with 20 ml of local anaesthetic in the form of 1% lignocaine with 1/200,000 adrenaline.

2 Incision and subplatysmal flaps
Using a 10 blade, incise through the skin and platysma, preserving the great auricular nerve and external jugular vein in the posterior part of the

Table 35.1: DEFINITIONS OF NECK DISSECTION

Type of neck dissection	Definition
Type I	Removal of all lymph node groups (levels I–V) with preservation of spinal accessory nerve (XI)
Type 2	Removal of all lymph node groups (levels I–V) with preservation of XI and the internal jugular vein
Type 3	Removal of all lymph node groups (levels I–V) with preservation of XI, intenal jugular vein and the sternocleidomastoid muscle
Supraomohyoid	Levels I–III
Antero-lateral	Levels I–IV
Lateral	Levels II–IV
Postero-lateral	II–V and also postauricular and suboccipital lymph nodes
Anterior/central	VI
Superior mediastinum	VII

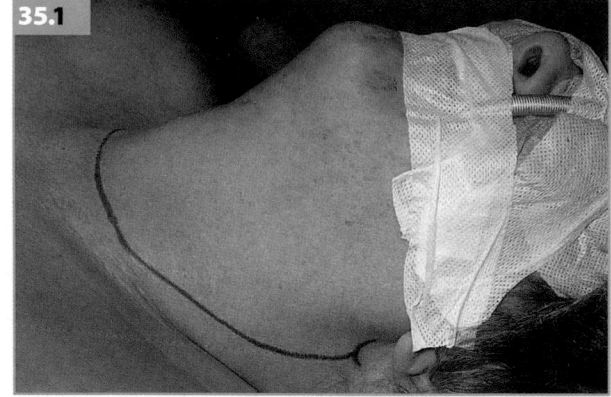

35.1 *Marking the incision.*

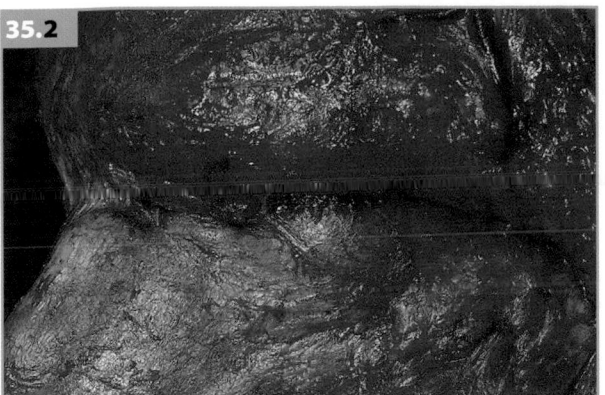

35.2 *Incision and subplatysmal flaps.*

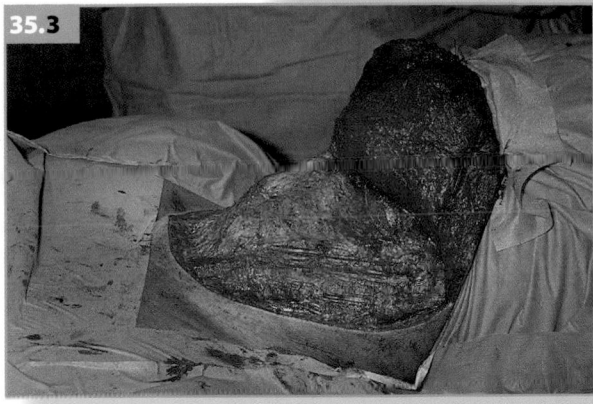

35.3 *Subplatysmal flaps.*

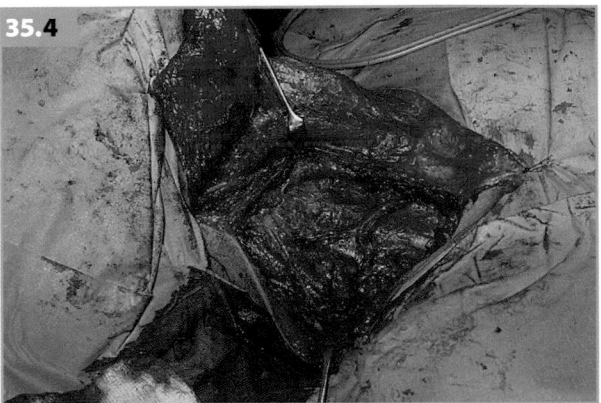

35.4 *Posterior flap.*

> ✪ **Surgeon's tip** _____
> *If exploring the neck for a deep space neck abscess, make an incision along the anterior border of the sternomastoid, and use blunt finger dissection to retract the sternomastoid and carotid sheath laterally, and thyroid and thyroid vessels medially, thus exposing the abscess and allowing drainage.*
> _____

incision. Ask your assistant to hold the skin flap under tension with catspaw retractors. Raise subplatysmal flaps, holding the blade parallel to the platysma and staying directly on the under surface of the muscle to avoid damage to the marginal mandibular nerve, which will lie deep to the flap (**35.2**).

Raise the flap superiorly as far as the border of the mandible. Raise the flap posteriorly as far as the sternocleidomastoid muscle. Use a stay suture to hold flaps in position and damp swabs to protect the flap (**35.3**).

If dissection of level V is required, dissection of the posterior skin flap should be extended as far as the trapezius muscle. When dissecting the skin flap posterior to the sternocleidomastoid, use your hand to hold the flap, and angle the knife parallel to the flap to protect XI, which runs very superficially in the roof of the posterior triangle (**35.4**). ✪

3 Level I

Identify the submandibular gland and marginal mandibular nerve running over its surface. Using a 15 blade, make an incision 2 fingers' breadth below the mandible through the fascia of the submandibular gland at its inferior edge, preserving the capsule to ensure oncological clearance. Elevate the fascia, again preserving the capsule, from the lateral aspect of the gland until you reach the superior edge. Beware of bleeding from the facial vein and artery.

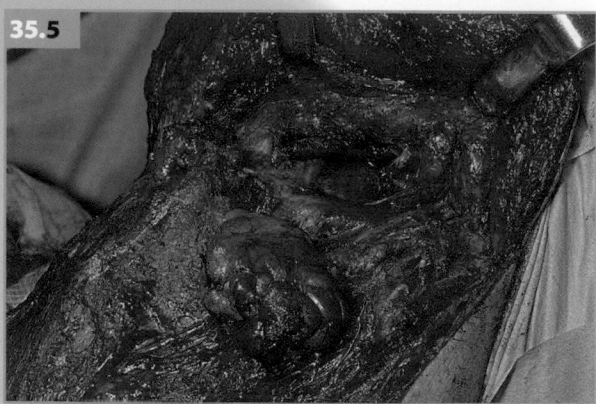

35.5 *Muscles are skeletonised.*

✪ **Surgeon's tip** _____
*The muscles of the floor of
the mouth and strap muscles
should be skeletonised during
your dissection, to ensure that
all the lymph nodes have been
removed (35.5).*

✪ **Surgeon's tip** _____
*By dissecting along the surface
of the bellies of digastric, you
avoid damaging the carotid
sheath, XI, and XII which lie deep
to the muscle.*

Divide and ligate the facial vein with 2/0 vicryl.
If possible, preserve the facial artery, in case it is
required for microvascular anastomosis. Retract the
mylohyoid anteriorly to expose the deep part of the
submandibular gland, lingual nerve, submandibular
ganglion, and submandibular duct. Ligate the
submandibular duct and dissect the deep part of
submandibular gland from the floor of the submandibular triangle.

Identify the anterior belly of digastric, and using
DeBakey forceps and McIndoe scissors dissect
forwards along the surface of the muscle until
you reach the submental triangle in the midline.
Using Allis forceps retract fibrofatty tissue off the
submental triangle, and continue the dissection
inferiorly towards the thyroid cartilage, staying in
the midline.

Using DeBakey forceps and McIndoe scissors
dissect posteriorly along the surface of the posterior
belly of digastric until you reach the mastoid tip. ✪

4 Identifying XI

Insert Langenbeck retractors, and retract the
sternocleidomastoid muscle posteriorly and the
posterior belly of digastric superiorly. Using a
mosquito clip held parallel to the direction of the
carotid sheath, gently divide the loose areolar tissue
overlying the cranial nerves and carotid sheath as
they exit the skull base. First identify the internal
jugular vein (IJV), and the upper sternomastoid
branch of the occipital artery which lies on its
surface. Divide and ligate this small artery to avoid
troublesome bleeding. Immediately below the
upper sternomastoid artery, and lying on the lateral
surface of the IJV, identify XI, and confirm this with a
nerve stimulator.

5 Level V

Just below the upper sternomastoid branch of the occipital artery, XI enters the sternomastoid muscle. Using a mosquito clip, follow the nerve through the body of the muscle until it divides into two branches, supplying the sternomastoid and trapezius. Follow the trapezius branch of XI as it leaves the posterior margin of the sternocleidomastoid muscle, approximately 1 cm below the great auricular nerve. Skeletonise the nerve as it traverses the roof of the posterior triangle. Use a mosquito clip to lift fibrofatty tissue off the nerve before dividing it, remembering that the course of the nerve becomes more superficial as it passes posteriorly. Hold the nerve out of the dissection field with a nerve sling.

Starting at the superior apex, clear the contents of the posterior triangle as far as the prevertebral fascia medially. Use Allis forceps to retract the fibrofatty tissue anteriorly, and skeletonise the prevertebral fascia using McIndoe scissors. Continue posteriorly as far as the anterior border of the trapezius. Inferiorly, the limit of the dissection lies at the superior edge of the clavicle. In order to prevent bleeding from the supraclavicular and transverse cervical vessels, use a large clip to divide and ligate the fibrofatty tissue of the inferior portion of level V in segments.

Continue dissecting anteriorly until you reach the carotid sheath (**35.6**). ✪✪

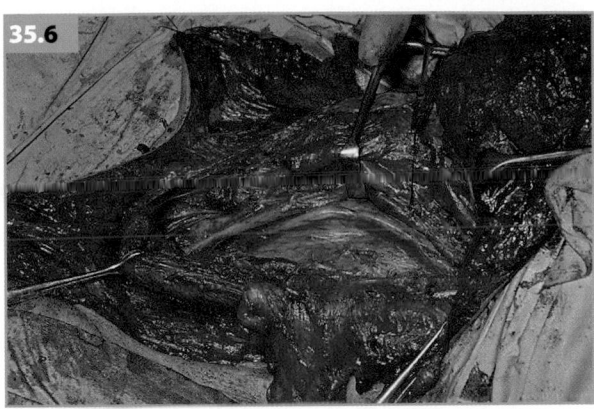

35.6 *Anterior dissection.*

6 Levels II, III, IV

Use a 15 blade to incise the fascia of the anterior border of the sternocleidomastoid muscle along its full length. Using Allis forceps, lift the fascia anteriorly and dissect it from the muscle fibres, until the underlying carotid sheath is fully exposed.

Using a 15 blade, dissect from the thyroid cartilage down to the sternal notch in the midline, and reflect fibrofatty tissue posteriorly. Identify the tendon of the omohyoid muscle where it crosses the IJV and divide using cutting diathermy.

> ✪✪ *Surgeon's tip* _____
> *The thoracic duct on the left, phrenic nerve, and brachial plexus lie deep to the prevertebral fascia and are protected from injury. Dissection deep to the prevertebral fascia is not normally necessary unless disease invades the fascia.*

Using McIndoe scissors, carefully open the anterior surface of the carotid sheath over the IJV, to avoid damaging X, which lies posteriorly. Open the carotid sheath along its whole length, ligating branches of IJV with 2/0 vicryl. Superiorly, just below the posterior belly of the digastric muscle, identify and preserve XII as it lies medially to IJV.

Join levels I, II, III, and IV with level V underneath the sternomastoid muscle, keeping the specimen en bloc (**35.7, 35.8**). ✪

7 Haemostasis, drains, and closure

Insert two size 16 drains, ensuring that they do not overlie the carotid sheath, and put the drains on suction while closing the wound. Use 2/0 vicryl to close the platysma and deep subcutaneous layer. Apply skin staples and a transparent dressing such as Tegaderm®.

8 Orientating the specimen

Using 16 G needles, pin the specimen onto a cork board, clearly marking levels of dissection. Alternatively, divide the specimen into separate levels, as agreed with your histology department.

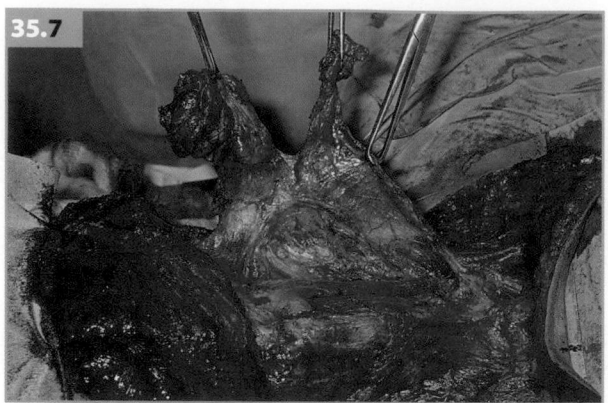

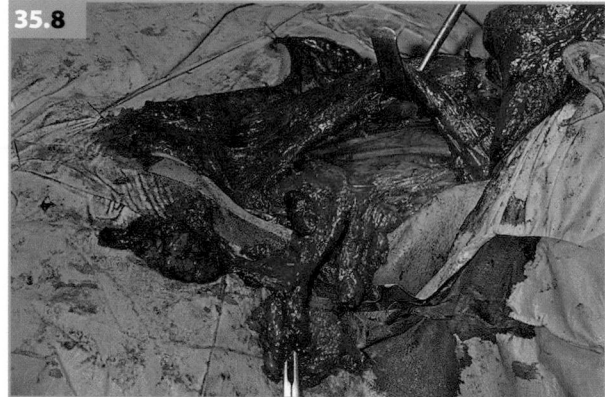

35.7, 35.8 *Join levels I, II, III, and IV with level V underneath the sternomastoid muscle.*

✪ *Surgeon's tip* _____
Level II is divided into IIa and IIb by the accessory nerve. It is important to include level IIb (which lies between the accessory nerve and skull base) in your dissection, as this is a common area for recurrent disease.

36 Total laryngectomy

SURGICAL STEPS

1 Positioning the patient
2 Confirming the diagnosis and stage
3 Incision and subplatysmal flaps
4 Dividing the strap muscles
5 Hemithyroidectomy
6 Dividing the suprahyoid muscles
7 Mobilising the larynx
8 Tracheostomy
9 Entering the pharynx
10 Laryngectomy
11 Cricopharyngeal myotomy
12 Primary tracheoesophageal puncture, speaking valve, and stomagastric tube
13 Closure of the neopharynx
14 Haemostasis, stomaplasty, and closure

PROCEDURE

1 Positioning the patient

Position the patient with a sandbag under the shoulders and a head ring, and the operating table head-up. Use a marker pen to indicate the line of incision, a Gluck Sorenson incision (**36.1**). Infiltrate with 20 ml of local anaesthetic in the form of 1% lignocaine with 1/200,000 adrenaline ✪

✪ *Surgeon's tip*

*If the laryngectomy is being performed with bilateral neck dissection, then the incision should run from the mastoid tip on one side, through the midline at a point half way between the cricoid and sternal notch, to the mastoid tip on the contralateral side (**36.1**, **36.2**). The neck dissection should be performed at the beginning of the procedure (see 35 – Neck dissection). If the laryngectomy is being performed without a neck dissection, the incision is smaller, and runs to the anterior border of sternocleidomastoid on each side, 2 cm below the angle of the mandible.*

2 Confirming the diagnosis and stage

Perform direct laryngoscopy to confirm the diagnosis, site, and stage of the tumour.

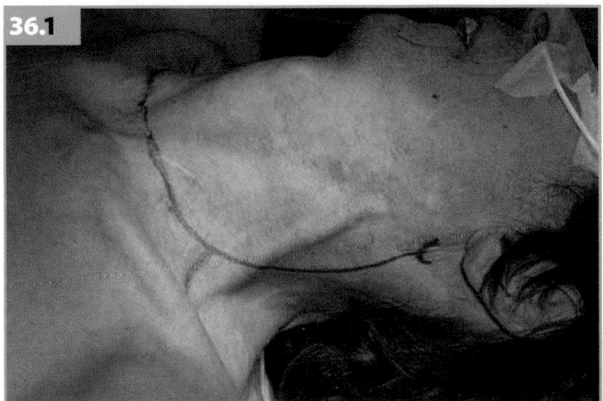

36.1 *Gluck Sorenson incision.*

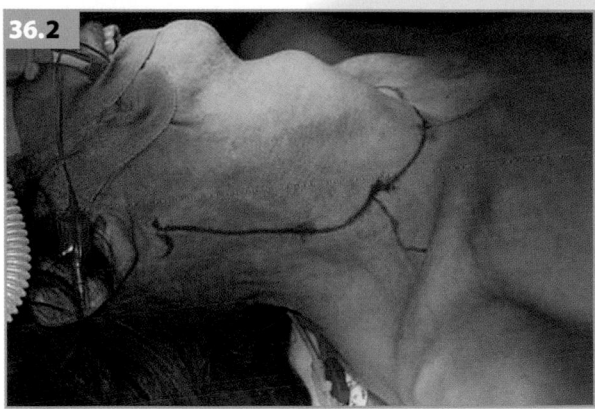

36.2 *Incision for bilateral neck dissection.*

36.3

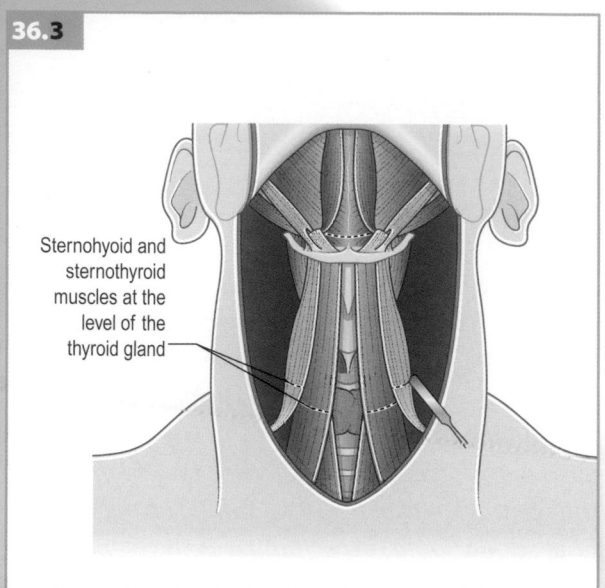

Sternohyoid and sternothyroid muscles at the level of the thyroid gland

36.3 *Dividing the sternohyoid and sternothyroid muscles.*

36.4

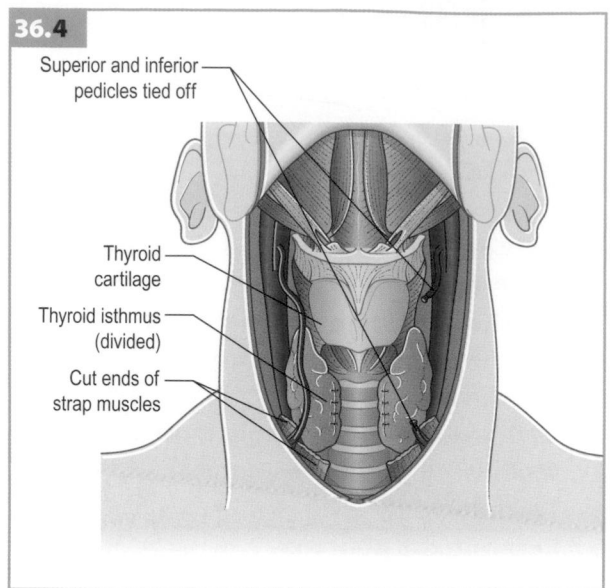

Superior and inferior pedicles tied off

Thyroid cartilage

Thyroid isthmus (divided)

Cut ends of strap muscles

36.4 *Dividing the thyroid isthmus and mobilising the thyroid.*

✪ Surgeon's tip

When mobilising the thyroid lobe which is to be preserved, take care not to traumatise the superior and inferior pedicles which supply the parathyroid glands.

3 Incision and subplatysmal flaps

Using a 10 blade, incise the skin, subcutaneous fat, and platysma. Ask your assistant to hold the superior skin flap under tension with catspaw retractors. Raise the subplatysmal flap holding the blade parallel to the platysma and staying directly on the undersurface of the muscle, to avoid damage to the marginal mandibular nerve and the anterior jugular veins which lie deep to the flap. Use 2/0 prolene stay sutures to hold the flaps in position, and damp swabs to protect the flaps.

4 Dividing the strap muscles

Using cutting diathermy, divide the sternohyoid and sternothyroid muscles at the level of the isthmus of the thyroid gland (**36.3**). Divide the omohyoid at its tendon.

5 Hemithyroidectomy

Hemithyroidectomy should be performed on the side of the tumour; where possible the contralateral thyroid lobe should be preserved. Divide the thyroid isthmus (*see 34 – Thyroidectomy*) and ligate the middle thyroid vein on the affected side. Identify and ligate the inferior and superior pedicles. Divide the recurrent laryngeal nerve. Leave the · hemithyroid attached to the trachea, and remove it en bloc with the laryngectomy specimen. On the contralateral side, dissect the thyroid lobe away from the trachea, and preserve it and the attached parathyroid glands (**36.4**). ✪

6 Dividing the suprahyoid muscles

Using cutting diathermy, divide the suprahyoid muscle attachments from the anterior border of the hyoid bone (**36.4**). Start in the midline and dissect laterally onto the greater cornu, to avoid inadvertently injuring the hypoglossal nerve. ✪✪

7 Mobilising the larynx

Using dissecting scissors, divide the pretracheal fascia to separate the carotid sheath from the lateral wall of the larynx on both sides. Continue dissection from the level of the trachea inferiorly to the level of the hyoid bone superiorly. Use cutting diathermy to skeletonise the thyroid cartilage. If possible, preserve the inferior constrictor muscle fibres to help reconstruct the neopharynx.

8 Tracheostomy

Aim to position the tracheostomy between the 2nd to 4th tracheal rings, but if the tumour is subglottic, then the tracheostomy will need to be placed lower than this. Use an 11 blade to enter the trachea, and continue the incision laterally onto the posterior wall of the trachea. Leave the posterior wall of the trachea intact at this stage. Insert a flexible tracheostomy tube (Rusch Montando tube) into the trachea, attach to ventilation, and suture the tube in place on the anterior chest wall (**36.5**). ✪✪✪

9 Entering the pharynx

Palpate the pre-epiglottic space to determine the level of the tip of the epiglottis. Use two pairs of Adson forceps to lift the mucosa of the pharynx on either side of the midline at this level. Use cutting diathermy to enter the pharynx in the midline, grasp the tip of the epiglottis with a Babcock forceps and retract anteriorly.

10 Laryngectomy

Using iris scissors, extend the incision laterally, along the aryepiglottic folds bilaterally. You now have a full view of the larynx and can assess the extent of the disease. Using iris scissors, continue the dissection inferiorly into the piriform fossa, if the disease permits. Place one finger inside the piriform fossa to stretch the mucosa and make dissection easier. Continue dissection posteriorly into the postcricoid region on both sides and mobilise the superior attachment of the larynx. Peel the larynx forward off the oesophagus as far as the tracheostomy inferiorly. You can now resect the posterior wall of the trachea. ✪✪✪✪

✪✪ *Surgeon's tip* _____
Rotate the laryngeal skeleton away from you in order to bring the greater cornu into view.

✪✪✪ *Surgeon's tip* _____
Warn the anaesthetist that you are about to perform the tracheostomy.

✪✪✪✪ *Surgeon's tip* _____
Preserving as much of the piriform fossa mucosa as possible allows pharyngeal closure without tension and reduces the risk of pharyngocutaneous fistula and stenosis.

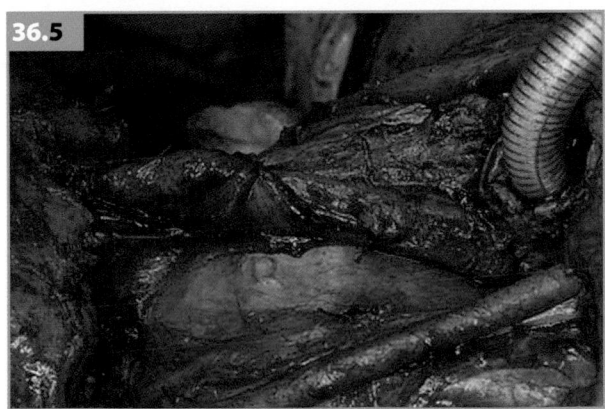

36.5 Tracheostomy.

11 Cricopharyngeal myotomy

Insert your index finger down the lumen of the oesophagus, and rotate the posterior aspect of the oesophagus into view. Using a fresh 15 blade, cut longitudinally down onto your finger, dividing first the longitudinal and then the circular oesophageal muscle fibres. Divide the last few fibres very carefully, to avoid perforating the oesophageal mucosa.

12 Primary tracheoesophageal puncture, speaking valve, and stomagastric tube

Insert a long curved forceps into the upper oesophagus and position the point of the forceps against the posterior wall of the trachea, in the midline, 1 cm below the edge of the tracheal stoma. Use a fresh 15 blade to cut down onto the tip of the forceps, dividing the trachea and oesophagus. Push the tip of the forceps through the hole, grasp the end of a size 16 stomagastric tube, and pull the tube back into the oesophagus. Push the tip down towards the stomach. Use a 2/0 silk suture to secure the stomagastric tube to the anterior chest wall.

13 Closure of the neopharynx

Use a 4/0 vicryl rapide to insert the first stitch at each end of the pharyngeal mucosa. Do not cut the suture, and leave the end of the suture long so you can put a mosquito clip on it. Your assistant gently lifts the suture at both ends to put the mucosal edge under tension. Then continue your running suture horizontally to the opposite side, making sure the suture everts the intraluminal mucosal edges.

Suture the inferior constrictor muscles together over your mucosal repair, to provide a second layer of closure.

14 Haemostasis, stomaplasty, and closure

Ask the anaesthetist to put the patient head down and normalise the blood pressure, to check for any bleeding. Insert two size 16 suction drains, making sure that the drain does not touch the anastomosis, and suture the drains in place with 2/0 prolene. Divide the stay sutures and trim the skin of the upper flap in a semi-circle around the tracheal stoma, so the skin is not under any tension. Use a 2/0 prolene to insert vertical mattress stitches between the skin and the tracheal edge, making sure that you do not leave any cartilage exposed.

Close the neck wound using 3/0 vicryl to platysma and deep subcutaneous tissues, and skin staples. Change the Rusch Montando tube to a double lumen nonfenestrated cuffed tracheostomy tube. Inflate the cuff, and suture the tube in position to avoid using tracheostomy tapes which may put pressure on the neck wound. ✪

✪ *Surgeon's tip* _____

An alternative technique for creation of the stoma is to fashion a separate incision in the lower flap, keeping the stoma separate from the Gluck Sorenson incision.

✪ *Surgeon's tip* _____

Divide the sternal heads of the sternocleidomastoid to avoid a depressed stoma.

37 Pectoralis major myocutaneous flap

SURGICAL STEPS

1 **Positioning the patient**
2 **Designing and marking the skin pedicle flap**
3 **Designing and marking the incision/ approach**
4 **Raising the skin pedicle**
5 **Delivering the pedicle to the neck**
6 **Closure**

PROCEDURE

1 Positioning the patient

The patient is positioned with a head ring and sand bag under the shoulders. The chest wall is prepared with betadine from the umbilicus to the clavicle.

2 Designing and marking the skin pedicle flap

Design your skin pedicle as shown (**37.1a, b**) in either a horizontal or vertical position. Avoid including the nipple as part of the pedicle as this will cause a poor cosmetic result. ✪

3 Designing and marking the incision/ approach

Mark the deltopectoral flap as shown (**37.2a**). For horizontal skin pedicles: connect the lower limb of the deltopectoral flap to the pedicle, using an incision along the anterior edge of the axillary fold (**37.2b**). For vertical skin pedicles: connect the lower limb of the deltopectoral flap to the pedicle with an incision across the chest wall as shown (**37.3**).

✪ Surgeon's tip

When determining the position of the pectoralis major flap, take into consideration, and therefore preserve, the possible future use of a deltopectoral flap as shown in **37.3**.

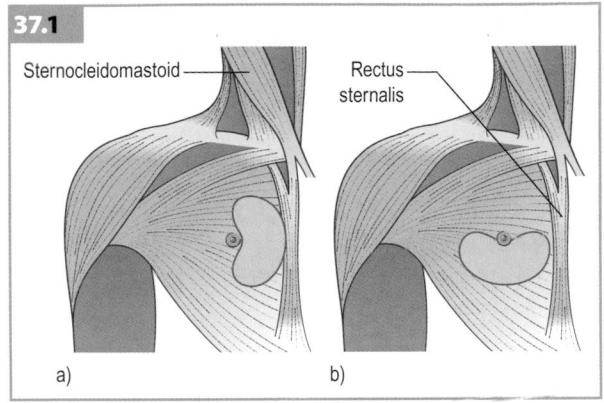

37.1 *Skin pedicle design.*

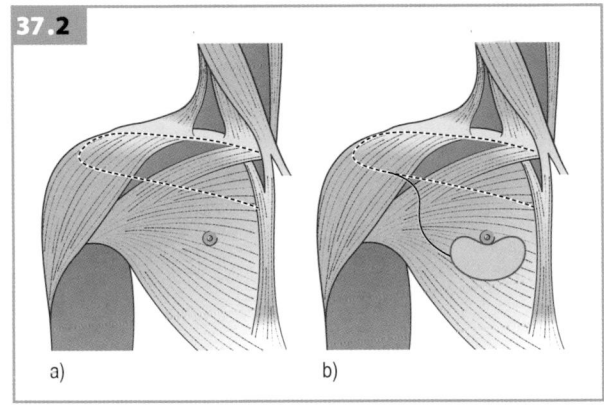

37.2 *Marking the deltopectoral flap.*

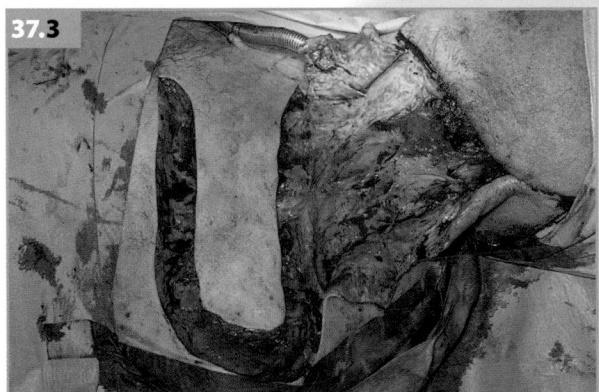

37.3 *Deltopectoral flap.*

4 Raising the skin pedicle

Make the skin pedicle incision using a 10 blade and incise the skin and subcutaneous fat as far as pectoralis fascia.

With a 3/0 vicryl suture, secure the edges of the skin pedicle to the pectoralis fascia to prevent shearing. Now connect the skin pedicle flap to the pectoralis flap with an incision through skin and subcutaneous fat as shown. Use McKindoe scissors to elevate the chest wall skin superior to the pedicle as far as the clavicle. Identify the pectoralis major muscle inferolaterally. Use finger dissection to delineate the plane between pectoralis major and minor muscles and separate the two. Now identify the pectoral branch of the thoracoacromial neurovascular pedicle which is the primary vascular supply for the flap.

Continuing with finger dissection, elevate the pectoralis major flap as far as the clavicle. Make sure you keep the neurovascular pedicle in view at all times and protect it from injury. As you dissect superiorly and approach the superior attachment of the pectoralis major to the clavicle, reduce the width of the flap (medial to lateral width) using McKindoe scissors. ✪

5 Delivering the pedicle to the neck

Once the pedicle is mobilised, create a small tunnel superficial to the clavicle into the neck. Use Babcock forceps to advance the flap back into the neck through the subcutaneous tunnel. Avoid twisting or occluding the vascular pedicle. ✪✪

6 Closure

A size 16 drain is inserted and the incision closed in two layers using 2/0 vicryl and skin clips.

✪ *Surgeon's tip* _____
Make sure your incision is slightly oblique to the fascia to include as many perforator vessels to the muscle as possible. This will maximise vascularity of the skin pedicle flap.

✪✪ *Surgeon's tip* _____
Free tissue transfer flaps are widely used as an alternative to the pectoralis major flap, e.g. radial forearm flap, antero-lateral thigh flap.

38 Local flaps

CONSIDERATIONS

- **Planning**
- **Z-plasty**
- **Advancement flap**
- **Bilobe flap**
- **Rhomboid flap**

Planning

Factors to consider when planning a local flap include:
- Site and size of defect (excision margin depends upon lesion pathology).
- Aesthetic units (**38.1**).
- Skin quality (patient age, smoker, scars, previous radiotherapy).
- Relaxed skin tension lines (RSTLs) (**38.2**).
- A variety of local flaps is available; the most common are described below.

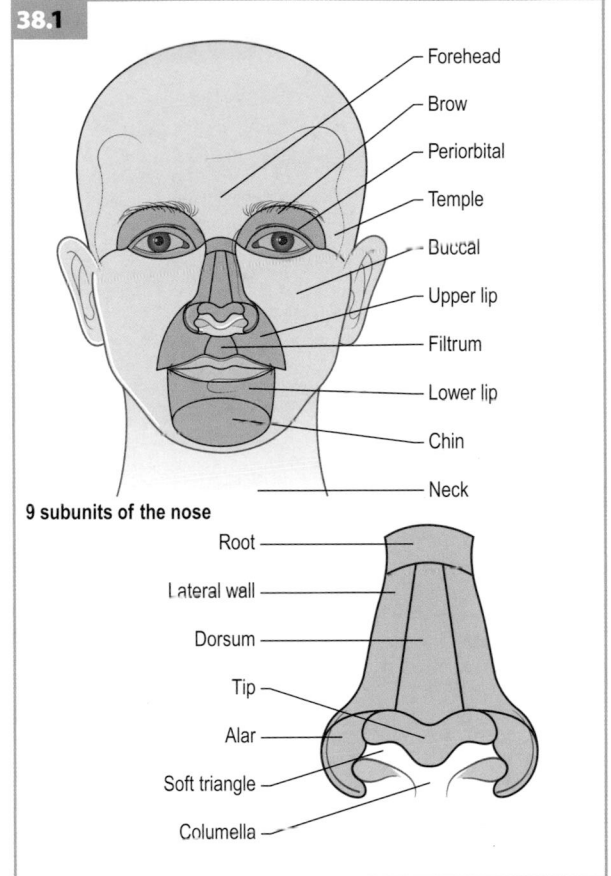

38.1 *Aesthetic units of the face.*

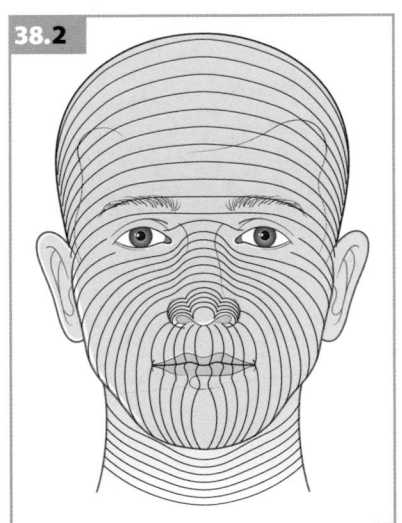

38.2 *Relaxed skin tension lines.*

Z-plasty

Use the Z-plasty to revise scars by increasing the length of the scar, reorientating the scar, or breaking up a straight scar.

SURGICAL STEPS

1 **Positioning the patient**
2 **Draping and local anaesthetic**
3 **Excision of the lesion**
4 **Raising local flaps**
5 **Closure and dressing**

PROCEDURE

1 Positioning the patient

Position the patient on a head ring, with the operating table head-up. Mark the extent of the lesion and excision margin. Design the flap, with two lines at angles of 60°, utilising RSTLs.

2 Draping and local anaesthetic

Use a head drape, and prepare the skin with betadine. If the procedure is being done under local anaesthetic, take care to leave the patient's eyes exposed. Inject subcutaneous local anaesthetic and adrenaline in the form of 2% lignocaine and 1/80,000 adrenaline to the planned incision site.

3 Excision of the lesion

Using a 15 blade, excise the scar. Ensure that the blade is held at right angles to the skin surface at all times, to avoid 'bevelling' the edge. Incise the limbs of the Z plasty.

4 Raising local flaps

Undermine the skin flaps so that sufficient skin is made available to transpose the tissue from A to B (**38.3**).

5 Closure and dressing

Suture points A to C and B to D using a 5/0 undyed vicryl (on the face) to anchor the flaps in position. Use 6/0 prolene to close the incisions, making sure to evert the skin edges and avoid closure under tension. Apply chloramphenicol ointment to the wound.

38.3

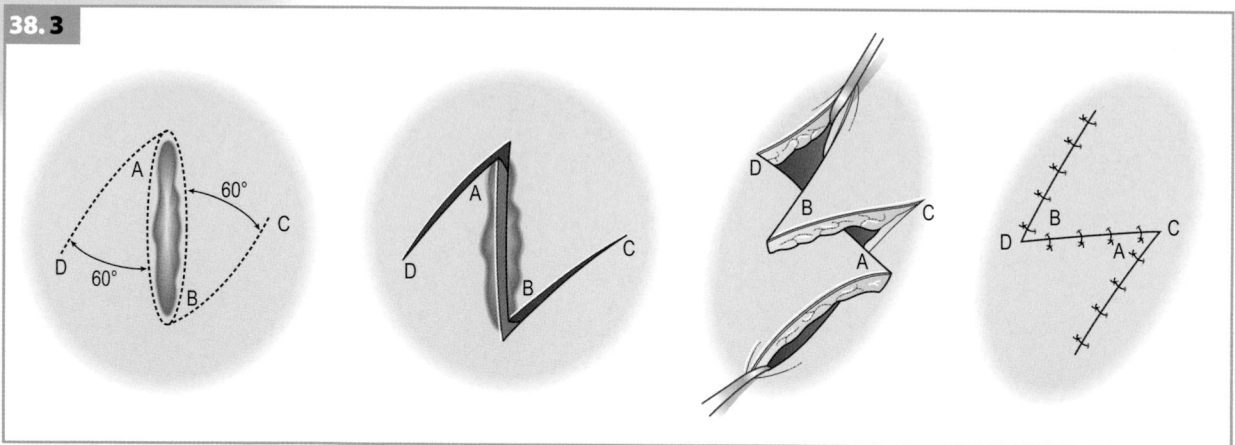

38.3 *Z-plasty.*

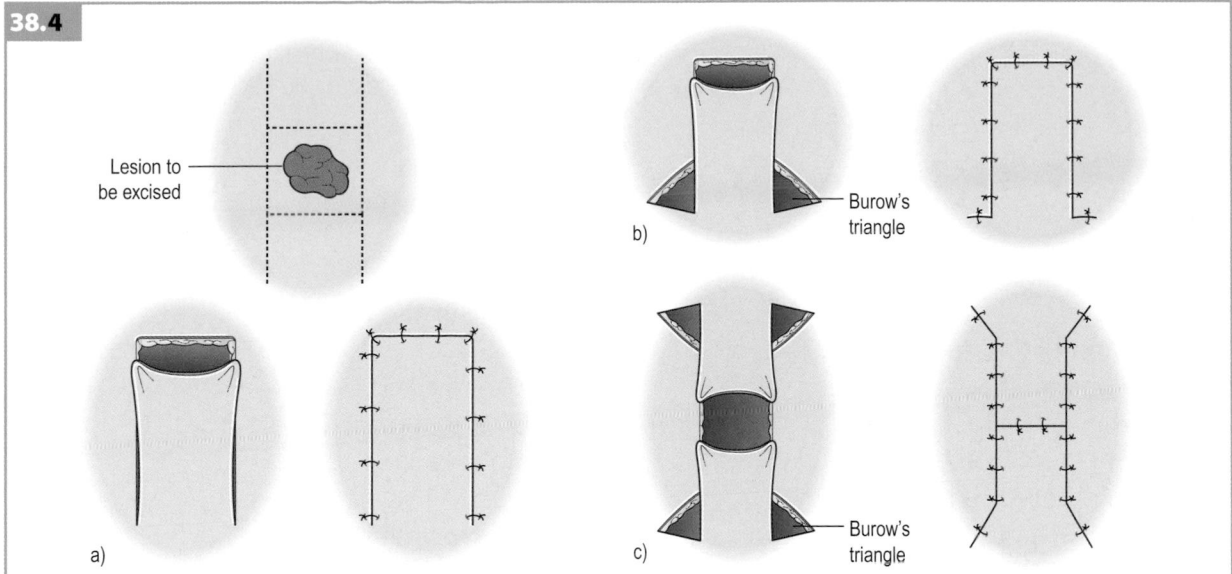

38.4 *Advancement flaps: a) advancement flap; b) with Burow's triangles; c) bilateral advancement flap.*

Advancement flap

Advancement flaps are used to advance tissue from one area to another. Burow's triangles may be used to bring in more tissue for advancement than a simple advancement flap alone.

SURGICAL STEPS

1   **Positioning the patient**
2   **Draping and local anaesthetic**
3   **Excision of the lesion**
4   **Raising local flaps**
5   **Closure and dressing**

PROCEDURE

1 Positioning the patient
Position the patient on a head ring, with the operating table head-up. Mark the extent of the lesion and excision margin. Design the flap, with Burow's triangles at the base of the flap if extra advancement is required (**38.4**). Bilateral advancement flaps can be used for larger lesions.

2 Draping and local anaesthetic
Use a head drape, and prepare the skin with betadine. If the procedure is being done under local anaesthetic, take care to leave the patient's eyes exposed. Inject subcutaneous local anaesthetic and adrenaline in the form of 2% lignocaine and 1/80,000 adrenaline to the planned incision site.

3 Excision of the lesion
Using a 15 blade, excise the lesion. Ensure that the blade is held at right angles to the skin surface at all times, to avoid 'bevelling' the edge. Incise the limbs of the advancement flap, and excise the tissue of Burow's triangles if necessary.

4 Raising local flaps
Undermine the skin flaps so that sufficient skin is made available to transpose the tissue into the defect.

5 Closure and dressing
Suture the 2 corners of the flap to the top of the defect using a 5/0 undyed vicryl (on the face) to anchor the flap in position. Use 6/0 prolene to close the incisions, making sure to evert the skin edges and avoid closure under tension. Apply chloramphenicol ointment to the wound.

Bilobe flap

Bilobe flap is a rotational flap, which advances tissue from adjacent skin areas, in a circular direction, by using two transposition flaps. It is very useful for filling defects on the side-wall of the nose.

SURGICAL STEPS

1 **Positioning the patient**
2 **Draping and local anaesthetic**
3 **Excision of the lesion**
4 **Raising local flaps**
5 **Closure and dressing**

PROCEDURE

1 Positioning the patient
Position the patient on a head ring, with the operating table head-up. Mark the extent of the lesion and excision margin. Design the flap, with two lobes as shown, with the base facing inferiorly to avoid flap oedema (**38.5**). If the lesion is on the side-wall of the nose, take care that your flap will not cause tension on the lower eyelid and produce an ectropion.

2 Draping and local anaesthetic
Use a head drape, and prepare the skin with betadine. If the procedure is being done under local anaesthetic, take care to leave the patient's eyes exposed. Inject subcutaneous local anaesthetic and adrenaline in the form of 2% lignocaine and 1/80,000 adrenaline to the planned incision site.

3 Excision of the lesion
Using a 15 blade, excise the lesion, and incise the skin flaps as marked. Ensure that the blade is held at right angles to the skin surface at all times, to avoid 'bevelling' the edge.

4 Raising local flaps
Undermine the skin flaps so that sufficient skin is made available to transpose the tissue from A to donor site, and B to A. Ensure adequate undermining so that defect b can be closed primarily.

5 Closure and dressing
Suture point A to primary defect, B to a, and b is closed primarily using a 5/0 undyed vicryl (on the face) to anchor the flaps in position. Use 6/0 prolene to close the incisions, making sure to evert the skin edges and avoid closure under tension. Apply chloramphenicol ointment to the wound.

Rhomboid flap

Rhomboid flap is a transposition flap with four limbs, which can be closed in a variety of different orientations. The donor site is closed primarily.

SURGICAL STEPS

1 **Positioning the patient**
2 **Draping and local anaesthetic**
3 **Excision of the lesion**
4 **Raising local flaps**
5 **Closure and dressing**

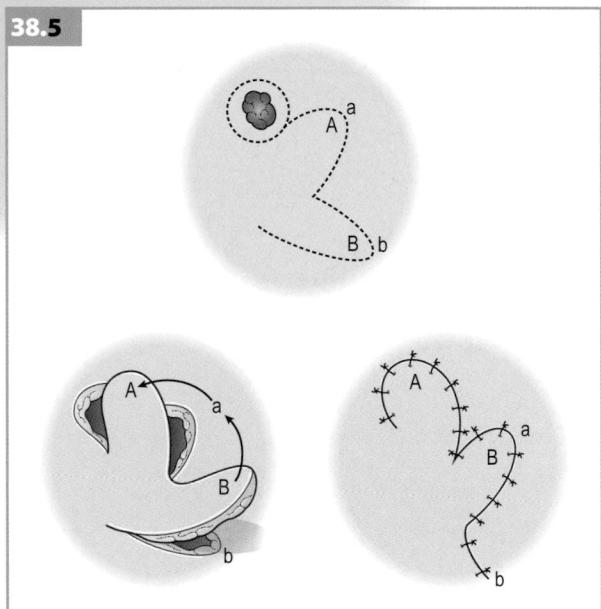

38.5

***38.5** Bilobe flap.*

PROCEDURE

1 Positioning the patient

Position the patient on a head ring with the operating table head-up. Mark the extent of the lesion and excision margin. Design a rhomboid flap around the planned excision margins, with angles of 60° and 120°. Mark a second rhomboid flap starting from the 120° angle of the first rhomboid, which will then transpose into the defect, as shown (**38.6**). The donor flap may be orientated in one of four ways in order to maximise RSTLs and skin availability.

2 Draping and local anaesthetic

Use a head drape, and prepare the skin with betadine. If the procedure is being done under local anaesthetic, take care to leave the patient's eyes exposed. Inject subcutaneous local anaesthetic and adrenaline in the form of 2% lignocaine and 1/80,000 adrenaline to the planned incision site.

3 Excision of the lesion

Using a 15 blade, excise the lesion, and incise the skin flaps as marked. Ensure that the blade is held at right angles to the skin surface at all times, to avoid 'bevelling' the edge.

4 Raising local flaps

Undermine the skin flaps so that sufficient skin is made available to transpose the tissue from A and B to donor site.

5 Closure and dressing

Suture points A and B to donor site using a 5/0 undyed vicryl (on the face) to anchor the flaps in position. Use 6/0 prolene to close the incisions, making sure to evert the skin edges and avoid closure under tension. Apply chloramphenicol ointment to the wound.

Also demonstrated in **38.7–38.9** is a V–Y advancement flap.

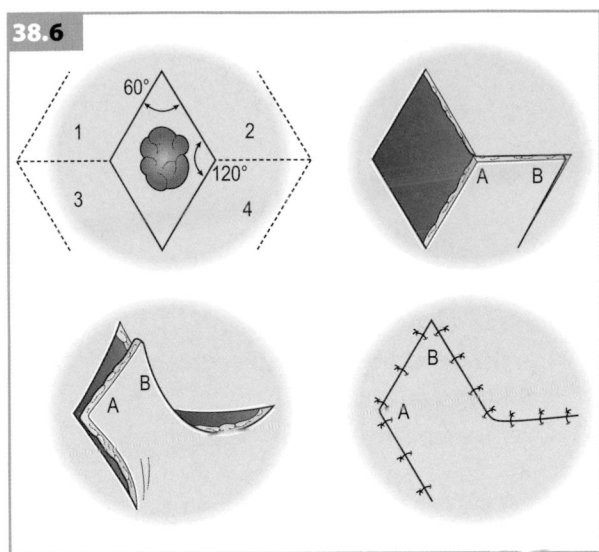

38.6 *Rhomboid flap.*

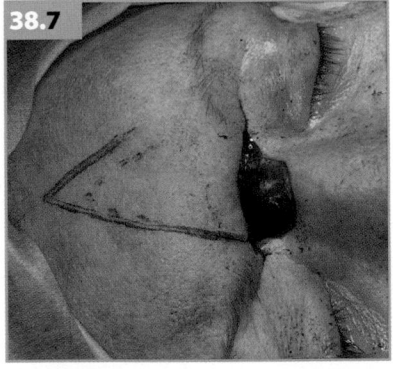
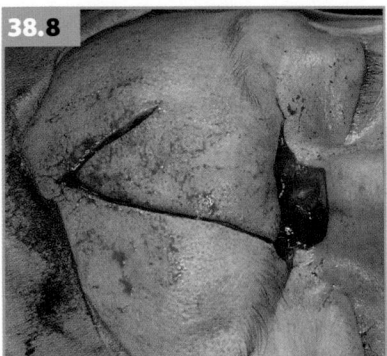
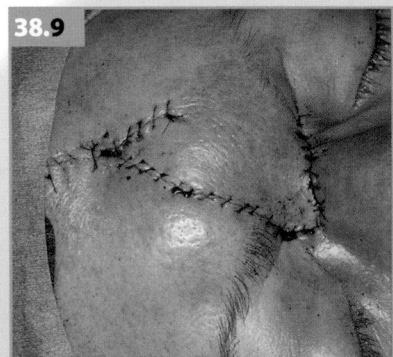

38.7–38.9 *V–Y advancement flap.*

39 Pinnaplasty

SURGICAL STEPS

1 **Positioning the patient**
2 **Marking and local anaesthetic**
3 **Postauricular incision**
4 **Cartilage exposure and scoring**
5 **Cartilage suturing**
6 **Closure and dressing**

PROCEDURE

1 Positioning the patient
Position the patient on a head ring with the operating table head-up. Turn the patient's head away from the operative side. A head dressing is used to cover the hair and a self-adhesive drape can be used to cover the whole face.

2 Marking and local anaesthetic
Using a sterile marker pen, mark the inferior crus, the superior crus, and the scapha as in Figure **39.1**. Use a 16G needle soaked in methylene blue to mark the planned convexity of both the superior crus and scapha (**39.2, 39.3**). Pass the needle through the pinna from anterior to posterior. Use capillary action to fill the lumen of the needle with dye, and then withdraw the needle through the cartilage, leaving a tattoo mark.

Inject 2 ml of local anaesthetic and adrenaline in the form of 2% lignocaine and 1/80,000 adrenaline using a dental syringe. Make sure the local anaesthetic is injected subperichondrially. Next, pull the pinna forward and draw an elliptical skin incision on the posterior aspect of the pinna (**39.4, 39.5**). Inject 2 ml of local anaesthetic and adrenaline.

3 Postauricular incision
Use a 15 blade to excise the marked ellipse of skin on the posterior aspect of the pinna down to the perichondrium. Remove any connective tissue and muscle on the postauricular sulcus down to the periosteum of the mastoid bone. Now dissect the skin anteriorly, towards the helix, until you reach the methylene blue markings (**39.6**). ✪

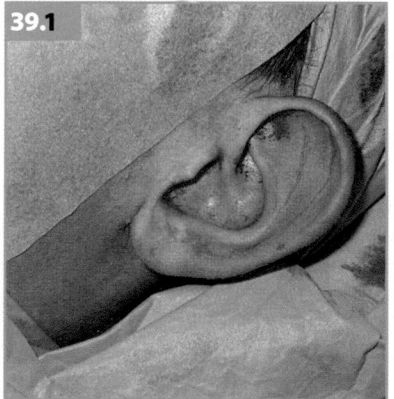

39.1 *Marking the inferior and superior crus and the scapha.*

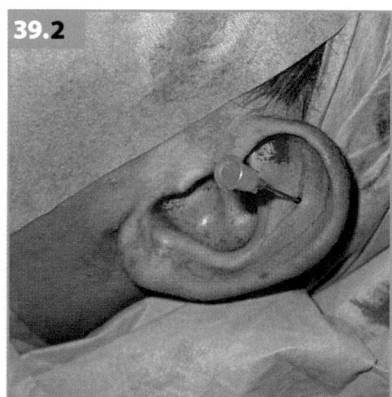

39.2, 39.3 *Marking the planned convexity of both the superior crus and scapha.*

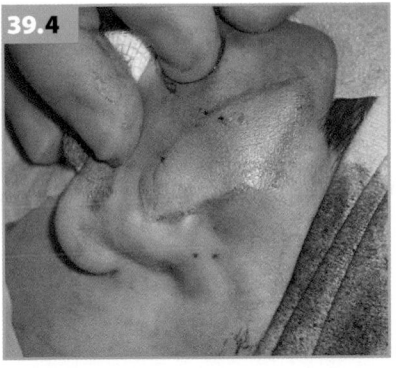

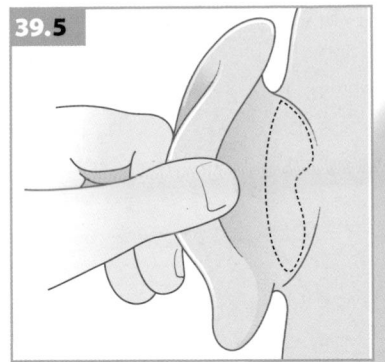

39.4, 39.5 *Marking the posterior skin incision.*

⚙ **Surgeon's tip** _____

Two main techniques are available for pinnaplasty – suturing and scoring. The traditional Mustarde technique uses conchoscaphal mattress suturing only.

_____

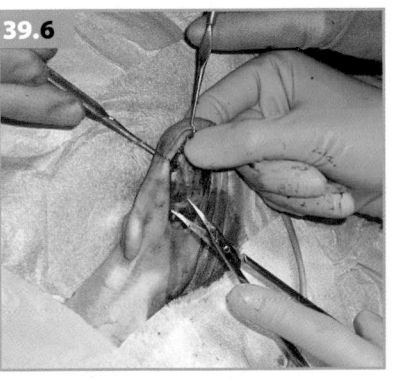

39.6 *Dissecting the skin anteriorly.*

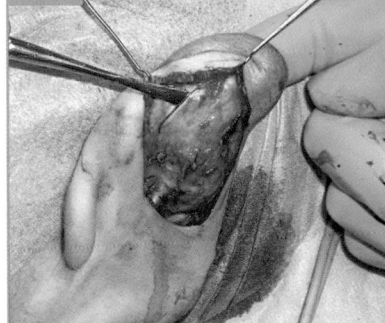

39.7 *Elevating the periosteum of the pinna anteriorly.*

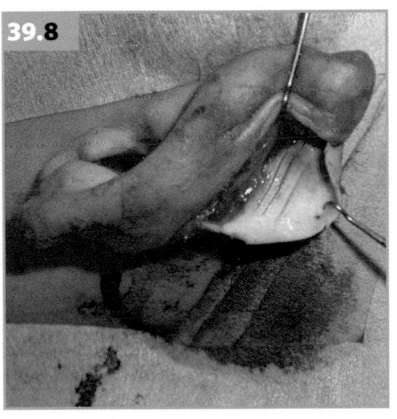

39.8 *Scoring the concave surface of the cartilage.*

4 Cartilage exposure and scoring

Using the 15 blade, incise the cartilage, taking care to avoid perforating the skin of the anterior surface of the pinna. Use a Freer elevator or curved iris scissors to elevate the periosteum of the pinna anteriorly as far as the whole length of the antihelix (**39.7**).

Use the 15 blade to score the concave surface of the cartilage (**39.8**).

5 Cartilage suturing

To create the antihelical fold, first assess the amount of folding necessary by furling the cartilage with index finger and thumb, then place a series of horizontal mattress sutures from the lateral aspect of the posterior pinna to the medial aspect. Place the superior suture first, followed by a further 3–4 mattress sutures as necessary (**39.9**, **39.10**). Only tie when all the sutures are in place, again starting with the superior most suture, adjusting the tightness to achieve the desired effect.

Finally, using a 4/0 absorbable suture, anchor the concha to the periosteum of mastoid bone to correct a deep conchal bowl (**39.11**).

6 Closure and dressing

Use a 4/0 prolene to close the postauricular incision. Measure the distance between pinna and mastoid bone (**39.12**) and follow the same procedure on the contralateral side. Make sure the distance on the two sides is the same for a symmetrical cosmetic result. Use a cotton wool ball to block the opening of the external ear canal; use a paraffin impregnated dressing such as Jelonet® to pack the concavities of the pinna and another Jelonet to cover the postauricular incision. Cover both ears with cotton wool and apply a head bandage. The head bandage should not be removed before 1 week postoperatively.

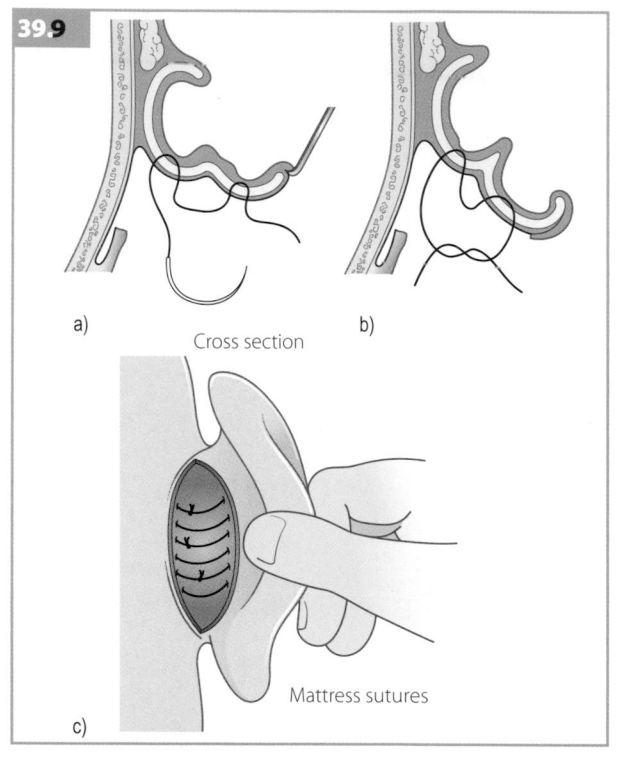

39.9

a)   b)

Cross section

Mattress sutures

c)

39.9 *Placing horizontal mattress sutures.*

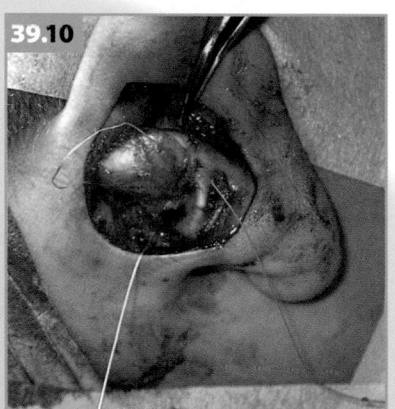

39.10

39.10 *Suturing.*

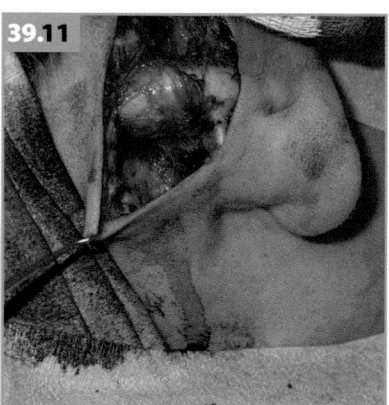

39.11

39.11 *Anchoring the concha to the periosteum of the mastoid bone.*

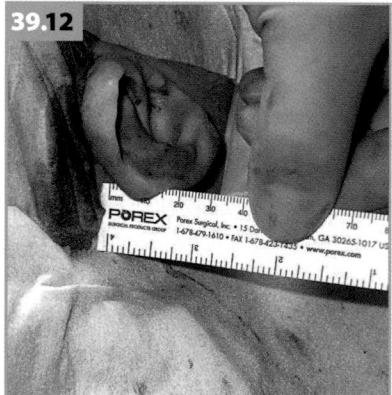

39.12

39.12 *Measuring the distance between the pinna and mastoid bone.*

40 Blepharoplasty

Upper eyelid

SURGICAL STEPS

1 **Preoperative marking**
2 **Positioning the patient**
3 **Skin incision**
4 **Resection of skin and muscle**
5 **Fat pad removal**
6 **Closure**

PROCEDURE

1 Preoperative marking

Mark the lower line of the incision on the superior tarsal border, which corresponds to the lower wrinkle of the upper eyelid. The scar will then lie in a natural skin crease. Mark the upper incision line according to how much excess skin and muscle needs to be removed. Remember to leave at least 2.5 cm of intact skin between the brow and eyelashes (**40.1**). The two lines meet medially just above the inner canthus and laterally along the crease of the upper eyelid. ✪

2 Positioning the patient

Position the patient on head ring (**40.2**). This procedure may be performed under local or general anaesthesia. Inject 2 ml of lignocaine with 1/80,000 adrenaline to the incision lines bilaterally. Use a dental syringe to inject the anaesthetic in the subcutaneous layer; avoid injecting anaesthetic into the globe.

3 Skin incision

Use a 15 blade to incise the skin under tension. Start at the medial end of the inferior incision, and continue to the lateral edge. Complete the incision along the superior margin, again starting medially and extending the incision laterally.

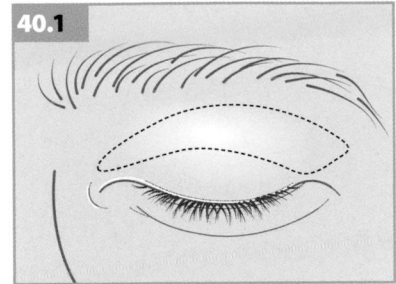

40.1 Marking the upper eyelid.

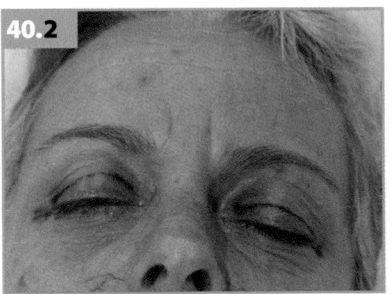

40.2 Marking the patient.

✪ *Surgeon's tip* _____
Make sure that you mark the incision with the patient in both supine and upright positions. Always remember that patients may have anatomical variations, and the eyes may not be symmetrical.

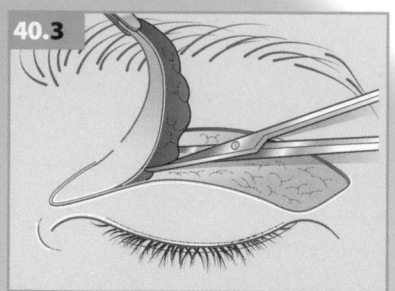

40.3 *Removal of skin and muscle.*

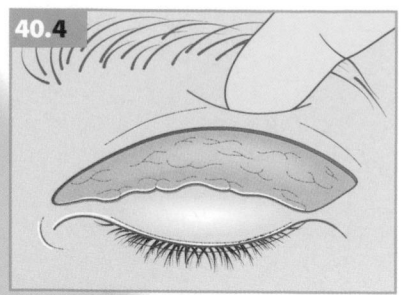

40.4 *Fat pad removal*

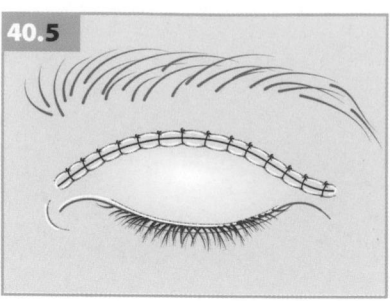

40.5 *Suturing.*

4 Resection of skin and muscle

Hold the skin with Adson forceps, and starting laterally excise the skin and orbicularis oculi muscle together. This releases the upper eyelid fat, which lies just beneath the muscle (**40.3**). If necessary, reduce the thickness of the lateral part of the orbicularis oculi muscle to reduce the chance of irregular or prominent scarring.

5 Fat pad removal

Incise the orbital septum, which lies beneath the orbicularis oculi muscle. Gently press the eyeball so that the fat pad herniates through the orbital septum (**40.4**). Hold the fat with two Adson forceps and use fine artery forceps to clamp the fat. Use monopolar cutting diathermy to remove the fat above the artery forceps. Release the artery forceps slowly, and use bipolar diathermy to cauterise any bleeding points. ✪

6 Closure

Using 6/0 prolene, close the muscle and skin edges laterally with two or three interrupted sutures. The remainder of the incision can be closed with a continuous 6/0 prolene suture (**40.5**). Apply ¼-inch steri-strips to the incision.

✪ Surgeon's tip _____

Incise the orbital septum from lateral to medial, taking care to avoid damaging the lacrimal sac medially.

Lower eyelid – transcutaneous approach

SURGICAL STEPS

1 **Preoperative marking**
2 **Positioning the patient**
3 **Skin incision**
4 **Fat pad removal**
5 **Resection of skin and muscle**
6 **Closure**

PROCEDURE

1 Preoperative marking

Mark the incision 2 mm below the tarsal margin (**40.6**). Medially the incision starts just below the lower punctum and extends laterally beyond the lateral canthus, following the natural skin crease for approximately 5–10 mm. This incision marking can be made with the patient supine.

2 Positioning the patient

Position the patient on a head ring. This procedure may be performed under local or general anaesthesia. Inject 2 ml of lignocaine with 1/80,000 adrenaline to the incision lines bilaterally. Use a dental syringe to inject the anaesthetic in the subcutaneous layer, avoid injecting anaesthetic into the globe.

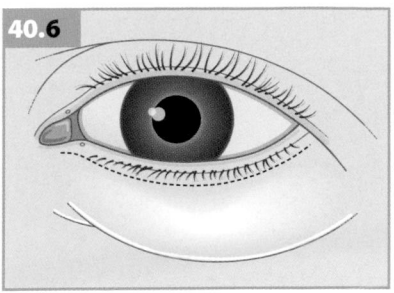

40.6 *Marking the lower eyelid.*

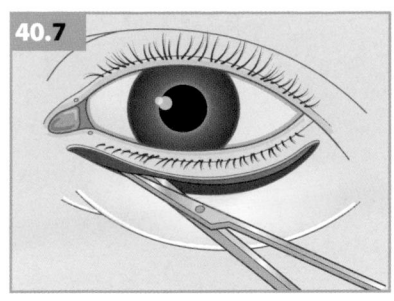

40.7 *Cutting the muscle along the line of the skin incision.*

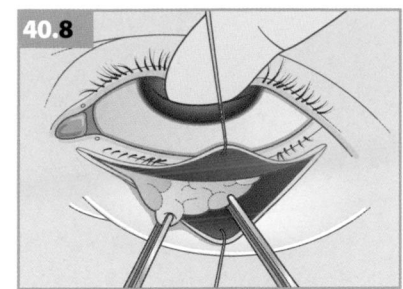

40.8 *Removing excess fat.*

3 Skin incision

Use a 15 blade to incise the skin under tension. Start at the medial end of the incision, ensuring that you only incise the skin, exposing the orbicularis oculi muscle. Using blunt iris scissors, cut through the muscle laterally and create a tunnel under the muscle (**40.7**). Use the scissors to cut the muscle along the line of the skin incision. Use two skin hooks to retract the lower eyelid superiorly and the skin and muscle inferiorly, to expose the medial aspect of the orbicularis muscle. Use a Lahey swab to develop a plane beneath the muscle, as far as the infraorbital rim.

4 Fat pad removal

Use Adson forceps to retract the medial fat pad and decide how much fat to excise. Hold the fat with two Adson forceps and use fine artery forceps to clamp the fat. Use monopolar cutting diathermy to remove the fat above the artery forceps (**40.8**). Release the artery forceps slowly, and use bipolar diathermy to cauterise any bleeding points. Usually, there is no need to reduce the lateral fat pad.

5 Resection of skin and muscle

If the orbicularis oculi muscle is hypertrophic, excise a narrow strip of muscle using iris scissors. Remove the excess skin, keeping the lower eyelid under tension and excising the skin from lateral to medial. Take great care to excise only a conservative amount of skin, especially medially, to avoid ectropion.

6 Closure

Use 6/0 prolene to close the skin edges laterally. Use two or three interrupted sutures to close the orbicularis muscle and skin together. Complete the closure with a continuous 6/0 prolene suture (**40.9**). Apply ¼-inch steri-strips to the incision.

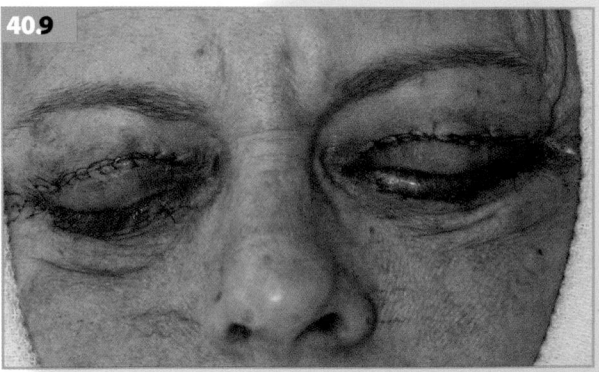

40.9 *Suturing.*

41 Face lift

SURGICAL STEPS

1 **Preoperative marking**
2 **Positioning the patient**
3 **Incision**
4 **Skin elevation and superficial musculo-aponeurotic system (SMAS) dissection**
5 **Submental dissection**
6 **Closure and dressing**

PROCEDURE

1 Preoperative marking

Mark the patient while in the upright position so that areas such as the jowls, nasolabial folds, and platysmal bands will be emphasised (**41.1**). Mark the following anatomical landmarks: angle of the mandible, jaw line, zygomatic arch, and the frontal branch of the facial nerve as it crosses the root of the zygoma.

2 Positioning the patient

Infiltrate the incision line and face with local anaesthetic and adrenaline. Minimise local anaesthetic toxicity with the tumescent technique – mix 100 ml of normal saline with 20 ml of 1% lignocaine with 1/200,000 adrenaline. Using a blue needle, infiltrate first the incision, and then change to a spinal needle and infiltrate the subcutaneous layer of the face and neck. ✪

3 Incision

The incision is divided into four parts – temporal, preauricular, postauricular, mastoid/occipital, and differs between males and females. In females the incision starts 2 cm above the tip of the pinna, behind the hairline and then joins the preauricular crease just above the tragus. The incision runs inferiorly across the posterior aspect of the tragus and then 2 mm anterior to the lobule as far as the insertion of the lobule. Continue the incision

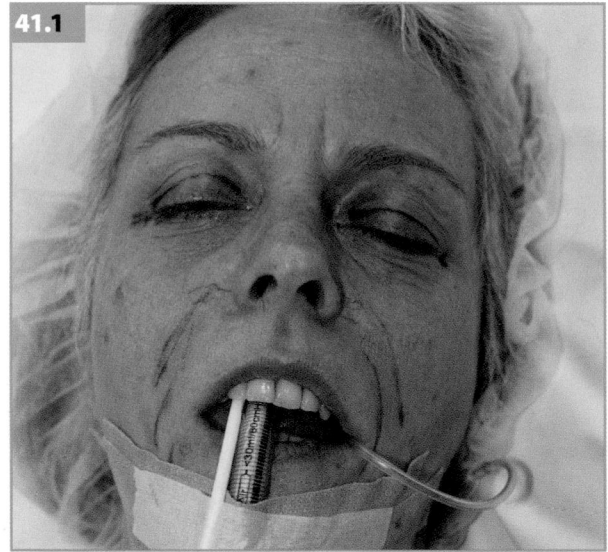

41.1 *Marking the patient.*

postero-superiorly in the postauricular sulcus as far as the level of the external auditory meatus. The incision then runs transversely across the mastoid and into the hairline. Follow the hairline inferiorly for 5–6 cm.

In males, the incision starts 2 cm above the tip of the pinna in the hairline, rather than behind it, then continues in front of the sideburn and turns posteriorly through 90° to a point 2–3 mm anterior to the ear lobule, before continuing as for females. This variation of the incision avoids the patient having hair-bearing skin over the tragus postoperatively or losing the sideburn. ✪✪

4 Skin elevation and SMAS dissection

Elevate the skin starting at the postauricular incision. The subcutaneous tissue is adherent to the sternomastoid fascia at its insertion to the mastoid tip. Dissect this carefully using a 15 blade until you reach the lateral border of the sternomastoid muscle. Continue the dissection in a subcutaneous plane anteroinferiorly as far as necessary (**41.2**). ✪✪✪ This dissection may connect with the dissection already made through the submental incision (*see step **5***).

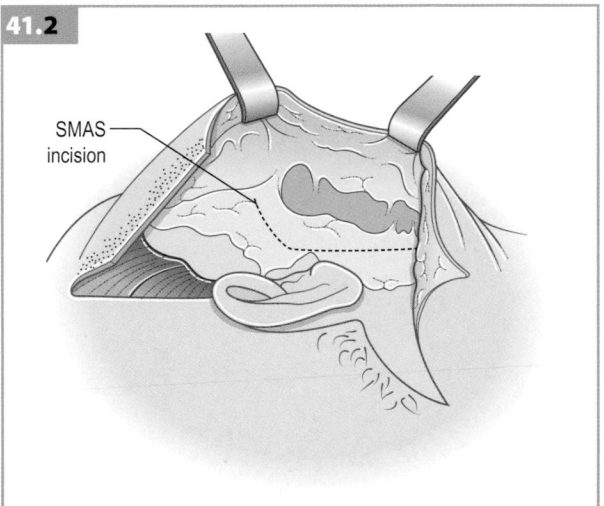

41.2

SMAS incision

41.2 *Incision of SMAS.*

Continue with elevation of the SMAS layer in the temporal region if necessary (when there is excess tissue at the side of the brow or in the orbital region). The dissection continues superiorly over the temporalis fascia, which fuses with the SMAS layer. The preauricular elevation is continued superiorly as far as just below the zygomatic arch superiorly and anteriorly as far as the insertion of the SMAS layer to skin.

Identify the SMAS layer anterior to the tragus, superficial to the parotid fascia. Dissect the sub-SMAS layer, on the deep surface of the SMAS, as far as the anterior border of the parotid. Insert two 3/0 prolene sutures, one superiorly from the SMAS to the temporalis fascia (**41.3**), and the other posteroinferiorly to the mastoid tip. These sutures provide vector retraction of the SMAS (**41.4**). ✪

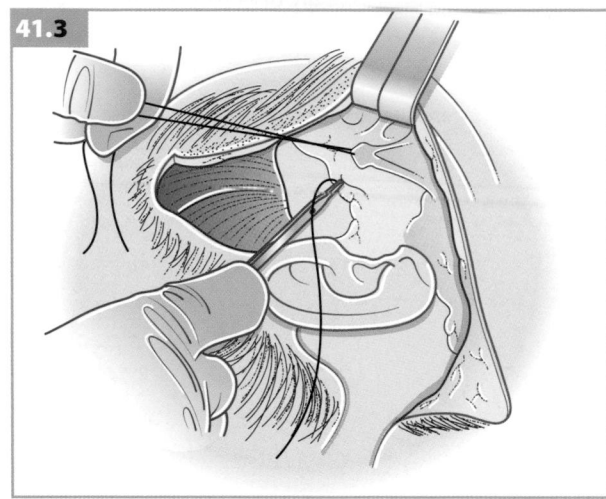

41.3 *Superior suture from the SMAS to the temporalis fascia.*

✪ **Surgeon's tip** ─────────
Take great care at this point of SMAS dissection, to avoid damaging the facial artery, vein, and the temporal branch of the facial nerve which lie on the lateral surface of the temporalis muscle.

✪ **Surgeon's tip** ─────────
Where there is a great deal of tissue to be retracted, excess SMAS layer may need to be trimmed before placing the vector sutures.

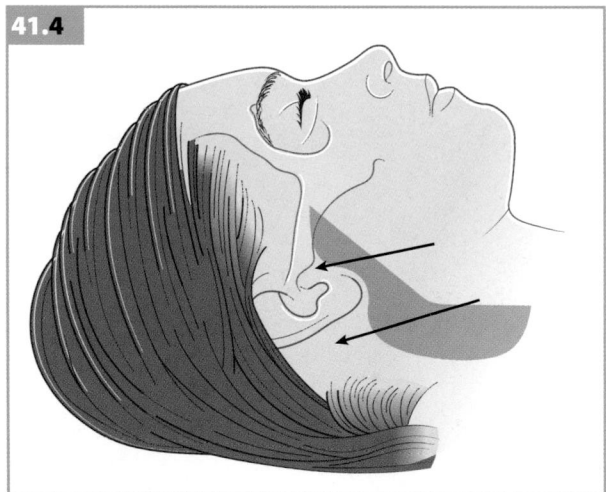

41.4 *Diagram to demonstrate vector retraction of the SMAS.*

5 Submental dissection

Using a 15 blade, make an incision along the submental skin crease to access the subcutaneous and submental fat in the midline of the neck. Remove the fat under direct vision using McIndoe scissors. Once the submental fat has been removed, suture the anterior borders of the platysma together using a 3/0 vicryl, to improve the cervicomental angle.

6 Closure and dressing

Remove any excess skin around the pinna (**41.5**). Retract the skin posteriorly and assess the amount of excess skin anterior to the pinna before excising it with McIndoe scissors. Then retract the post-auricular skin in a superior direction, and excise any redundant skin (**41.6**). Insert a size 8 redivac drain.

Avoid tension along the skin edges to prevent unsightly scarring. Close the deep subcutaneous layer with interrupted 4/0 undyed vicryl. For skin, use 6/0 prolene for the preauricular part of the incision, 5/0 prolene for the postauricular part, and skin clips for the hair-bearing part (**41.7**).

Apply a pressure bandage for 24 hours (**41.8**).

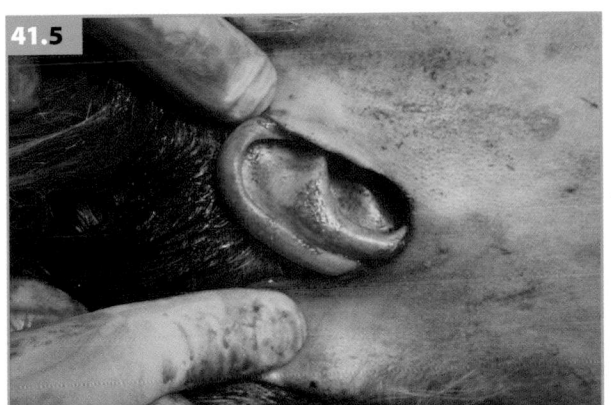

41.5 *Removing excess skin from around the pinna.*

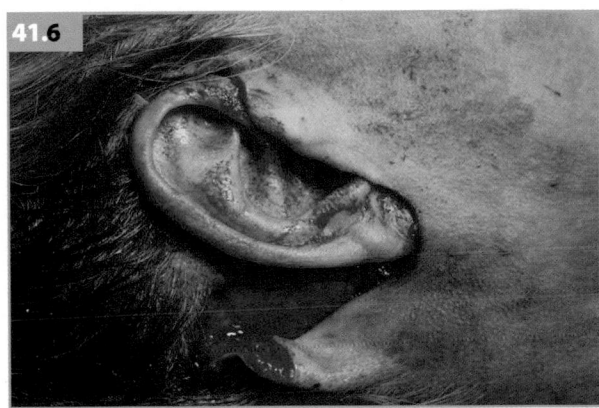

41.6 *Retracting the postauricular skin in a superior direction, and excising any redundant skin.*

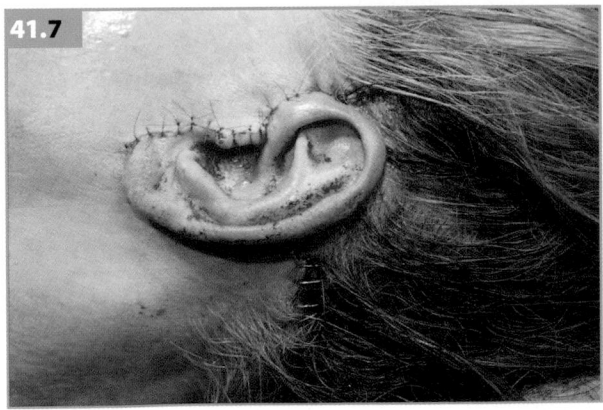

41.7 *Skin sutures and clips.*

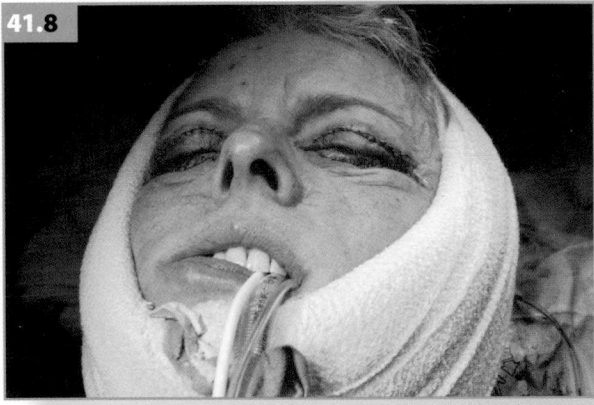

41.8 *Pressure bandage.*

Index